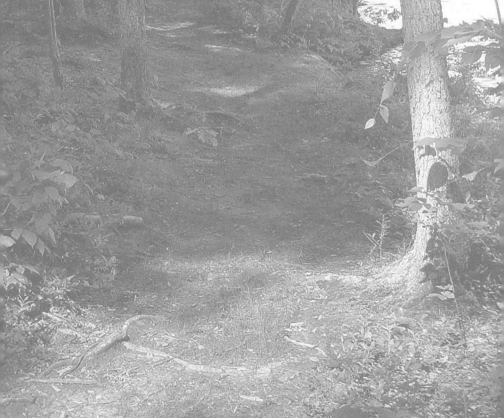

The Official
Rails-to-Trails
Conservancy
Guidebook

Rail-Trails
Mid-Atlantic

Rail-Trails: Mid-Atlantic

1st EDITION January 2007
7th printing 2013

Copyright © 2007 by Rails-to-Trails Conservancy

Front and back cover photographs copyright © 2007 by Alicia F. Klenk
(front, main image); Duncan Haas *(front, upper left)*; Corey Hilz
(front, lower right); and Rails-to-Trails Conservancy *(back)*
Photograph on p. 93 by Sally Olds; p. 111 by Jim Wyman
All other interior photographs by Rails-to-Trails Conservancy

Maps: Gene Olig and Lohnes+Wright

Map data courtesy of: Environmental Systems Research Institute
Cover design: Lisa Pletka and Barbara Richey
Book design and layout: Lisa Pletka
Book editors: Karen Stewart, Jennifer Kaleba, and Eva Dienel

ISBN: 978-0-89997-427-9

Manufactured in the United States of America

Published by: **Wilderness Press**
Keen Communications
PO Box 43673
Birmingham, AL 35243
(800) 443-7227
info@wildernesspress.com
www.wildernesspress.com

Visit our website for a complete listing of our books and for ordering
information.

Distributed by Publishers Group West

Cover photos: New River Trail *(main image)*;
Virginia Creeper National Recreation Trail *(upper left)*; Number
Nine Trolly Line *(lower right)*; Patuxent Branch Trail *(back cover)*

Title page photo: Railroad Ford Trail

About Rails-to-Trails Conservancy

Headquartered in Washington, DC, Rails-to-Trails Conservancy (RTC) fosters one great mission: to protect America's irreplaceable rail corridors by transforming them into multiuse trails. Its hope is that these pathways will reconnect Americans with their neighbors, communities, nature, and proud history.

Railways helped build America. Spanning from coast to coast, these ribbons of steel linked people, communities, and enterprises, spurring commerce and forging a single nation that bridges a continent. But in recent decades, many of these routes have fallen into disuse, severing communal ties that helped bind Americans together.

When RTC opened its doors in 1986, the rail-trail movement was in its infancy. While there were some 250 miles of open rail-trails in the United States, most projects focused on single, linear routes in rural areas, created for recreation and conservation. RTC sought broader protection for the unused corridors, incorporating rural, suburban, and urban routes.

Year after year, RTC's efforts to protect and align public funding with trail building created an environment that allowed trail advocates in communities all across the country to initiate trail projects. These ever-growing ranks of trail professionals, volunteers, and RTC supporters have built momentum for the national rail-trails movement. As the number of supporters multiplied, so too did the rail-trails. By the turn of the 21st century, there were some 1100 rail-trails on the ground, and RTC recorded nearly 84,000 supporters, from business leaders and politicians to environmentalists and healthy-living advocates.

Americans now enjoy more than 13,000 miles of open rail-trails. And as they flock to the trails to commune with neighbors, neighborhoods, and nature, their economic, physical, and environmental wellness continues to flourish.

In 2006, Rails-to-Trails Conservancy celebrated 20 years of creating, protecting, serving, and connecting rail-trails. Boasting more than 100,000 members and supporters, RTC is the nation's leading advocate for trails and greenways.

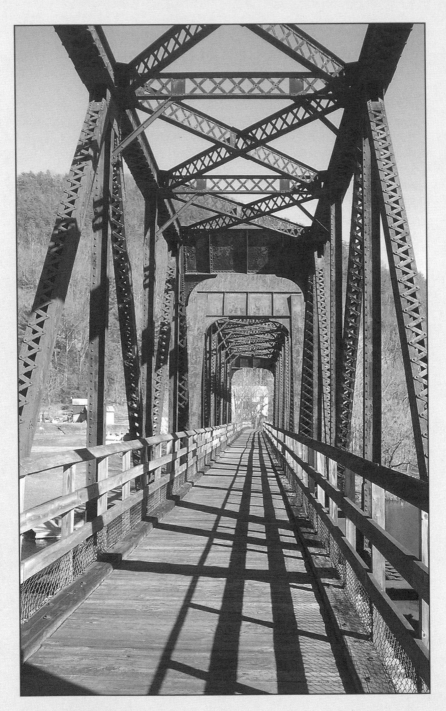

New River Trail State Park, Virginia

Foreword

Dear Reader:

First, for those of you who have already experienced the sheer enjoyment and freedom of riding on a rail-trail, welcome back! You'll find *Rail-Trails: Mid-Atlantic* to be a useful and fun guide to your favorite trails. It may even help you find some new pathways you didn't already know about.

For you readers who are discovering, for the first time, the adventures you can have on a rail-trail, thank you for joining the rail-trail movement. Since 1986, Rails-to-Trails Conservancy has been the No. 1 supporter and defender of these priceless public corridors, and we are excited to bring you *Rail-Trails: Mid-Atlantic* so you, too, can enjoy this region's rail-trails.

Built on unused, former railroad corridors, these hiking and biking trails are ideal ways to connect with your community, with nature, and with your friends and family. I've found that rail-trails have a way of bringing people together, and as you'll see from this book, you have opportunities in every state you visit to get on a trail. Whether you're looking for a place to exercise, explore, commute, or play—there is a rail-trail in this book for you.

So I invite you to sit back, relax, pick a trail that piques your interest—and then get out, get active, and have some fun. I'll be out on the trails, too, so be sure to wave as you go by.

Happy Trails,
Keith Laughlin
President, Rails-to-Trails Conservancy

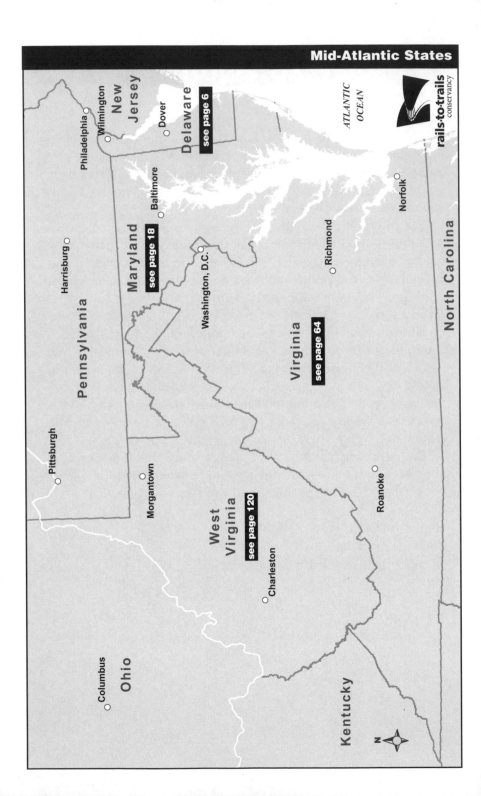

Mid-Atlantic States

rails·to·trails
conservancy

*ATLANTIC
OCEAN*

New Jersey

Wilmington

Philadelphia

Dover

Delaware
see page 6

Baltimore

Norfolk

Harrisburg

Maryland
see page 18

Richmond

Pennsylvania

Washington, D.C.

Virginia
see page 64

North Carolina

Pittsburgh

Morgantown

West
Virginia
see page 120

Roanoke

Columbus

Ohio

Charleston

Kentucky

N

Contents

DELAWARE   6

MARYLAND   18

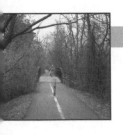

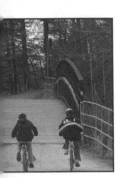

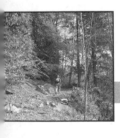

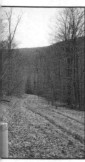

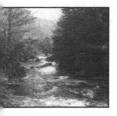

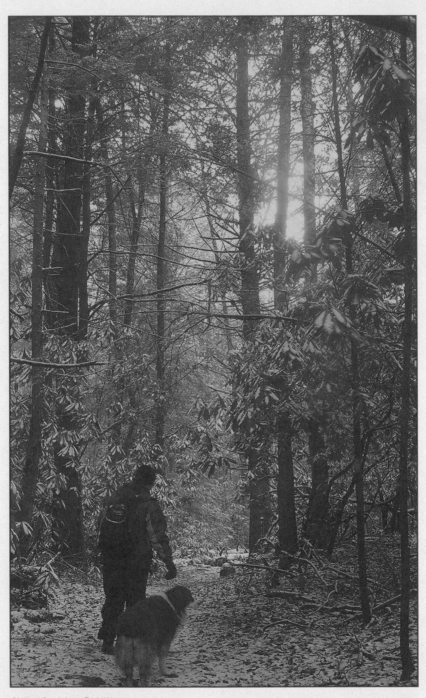

Phillips Creek Loop Trail, Virginia

INTRODUCTION

O f the more than 1400 rail-trails across the US, 112 thread through the Mid-Atlantic states of Delaware, Maryland, Virginia, and West Virginia. These routes relate a two-part story: The first speaks to the early years of railroading, while the second showcases efforts by Rails-to-Trails Conservancy, other groups, and their supporters to resurrect these unused railroad corridors as public-use trails.

Rail-Trails: Mid-Atlantic highlights 56 of the region's diverse trails, each serving as a window into the communities the railroad once served. Some trails delve into the particular history of an area, such as Virginia's Hanging Rock Battlefield Trail, which tells of Civil War battles and the importance of the railroad to the troops. Other trails tell a more docile tale, such as Maryland's Savage Mill Trail. At its trailhead stands a renovated 1822 textile mill.

With the most trails of the region, West Virginia also boasts some of the most rural and unique rail-trails. Not always the flat and even pathways you might expect from rail-trails, West Virginia's trails offer a variety of backwoods treks such as the Limerock and Otter Creek Wilderness trails of the Monongahela National Forest. To compliment these rustic pathways are the well-groomed yet still wild and wonderful Mountain State trails like the gorgeous and popular 77-mile Greenbrier River Trail, or the paved, city trails of Morgantown.

Next door, Virginia is also a keeper of rail-trail gems. No guide to the area would be complete without featuring the state's southern Virginia Creeper National Recreation Trail or New River Trail. In the northern part of the state, right outside the bustle of Washington, DC, the Washington and Old Dominion Railroad Regional Park takes riders out of the city and into rolling farmland and horse country.

Washington, DC, itself is home to a portion of the Capital Crescent Trail, which begins in suburban Maryland before heading to the historical and trendy Georgetown neighborhood. And in the state best known for its crabs and waterways, Maryland's Cross Island Trail is a coastal sojourn. The only closer you could get would be to meander on Delaware's Junction and Breakwater Trail, which sits in the heart of the state's recreational beach area.

No matter which route in *Rail-Trails: Mid-Atlantic* you decide to try, you'll be touching on the heart of the community that helped build it and the history that first brought the rails to the region.

What is a Rail-Trail?

Rail-trails are multiuse public paths built along former railroad corridors. Most often flat or following a gentle grade, they are suited to walking, running, cycling, mountain biking, inline skating, cross-country skiing, horseback riding, and wheelchair use. Since the 1960s, Americans have created more than 13,000 miles of rail-trails throughout the country.

These extremely popular recreation and transportation corridors traverse urban, suburban, and rural landscapes. Many preserve historic landmarks, while others serve as wildlife conservation corridors, linking isolated parks and establishing greenways in developed areas. Rail-trails also stimulate local economies by boosting tourism and promoting trailside businesses.

What is a Rail-with-Trail?

A rail-with-trail is a public path that parallels a still-active rail line. Some run adjacent to high-speed, scheduled trains, often linking public transportation stations, while others follow tourist routes and slow-moving excursion trains. Many share an easement, separated from the rails by extensive fencing. There are more than 115 rails-with-trails in the US.

HOW TO USE THIS BOOK

*R*ail-Trails: Mid-Atlantic provides the information you'll need to plan a rewarding rail-trail trek. With words to inspire you and maps to chart your path, it makes choosing the best route a breeze. Following are some of the highlights.

Maps

You'll find three levels of maps in this book: an **overall regional map**, **state locator maps**, and **detailed trail maps**.

The Mid-Atlantic region includes Delaware, Maryland, Virginia, and West Virginia. Each chapter details a particular state's network of trails, marked on locator maps in the chapter introduction. Use these maps to find the trails nearest you, or select several neighboring trails and plan a weekend hiking or biking excursion. Once you find a trail on a state locator map, simply flip to the corresponding page number for a full description. Accompanying trail maps mark each route's access roads, trailheads, parking areas, restrooms, and other defining features.

Regional map

State locator map

Trail map

3

Trail Descriptions

Trails are listed in alphabetical order within each chapter. Each description leads off with a set of summary information, including trail endpoints and mileage, a roughness index, the trail surface, and possible uses.

The map and summary information list the trail endpoints (either a city, street, or more specific location), with suggested points from which to start and finish. Additional access points are marked on the maps and mentioned in the trail descriptions. The maps and descriptions also highlight available amenities, including parking and restrooms, as well as such area attractions as shops, services, museums, parks, and stadiums. Trail length is listed in miles.

Each trail bears a roughness index rating from 1 to 3. A rating of 1 indicates a smooth, level surface that is accessible to users of all ages and abilities. A 2 rating means the surface may be loose and/or uneven and could pose a problem for road bikes and wheelchairs. A 3 rating suggests a rough surface that is only recommended for mountain bikers and hikers. Surfaces can range from asphalt or concrete to ballast, cinder, crushed stone, gravel, grass, dirt, and/or sand. Where relevant, trail descriptions address alternating surface conditions.

All rail-trails are open to pedestrians, and most allow bicycles, except where noted in the trail summary or description. The summary also indicates wheelchair access. Other possible uses include inline skating, mountain biking, hiking, horseback riding, fishing, and cross-country skiing. While most trails are off-limits to motor vehicles, some local trail organizations do allow ATVs and snowmobiles.

Trail descriptions themselves suggest an ideal itinerary for each route, including the best parking areas and access points, where to begin, your direction of travel, and any highlights along the way. The text notes any connecting or neighboring routes, with page numbers for the respective trail descriptions. Following each description are directions to the recommended trailheads.

Each trail description also lists a local contact (name, address, phone number, and website) for further information. Be sure to call these trail managers or volunteer groups in advance for updates and current conditions.

Key to Map Icons

Parking   **Drinking water**   **Bathrooms**

Trail Use

Rail-trails are popular routes for a range of uses, often making them busy places to play. Trail etiquette applies. If passing other trail users on your bicycle, always try to pass on the left with an audible warning such as a bike-mounted bell or a polite but firm, "Passing on your left!" For your safety and that of other trail users, keep children and pets from straying into oncoming trail traffic. Keep dogs leashed, and supervise children until they can demonstrate proper behavior.

Cyclists and inline skaters should wear helmets, reflective clothing, and other safety gear, as some trails involve hazardous road crossings. It's also best to bring a flashlight or bike- or helmet-mounted light for tunnel passages or twilight excursions.

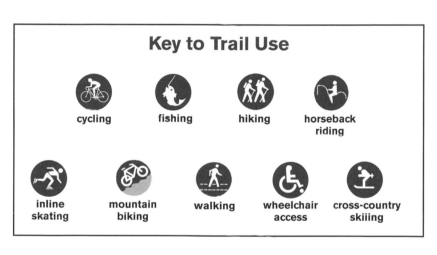

Key to Trail Use

cycling   fishing   hiking   horseback riding

inline skating   mountain biking   walking   wheelchair access   cross-country skiing

Learn More

While *Rail-Trails: Mid-Atlantic* is a helpful guide to available routes in the region, it wasn't feasible to list every rail-trail in the Mid-Atlantic, and new rail-trails spring up each year. To learn about additional rail-trails in your area or to plan a trip to an area beyond the scope of this book, log on to the Rails-to-Trails Conservancy home page (www.railstotrails.org) and click on the Find a Trail link. RTC's online database lists more than 1400 rail-trails nationwide, searchable by state, county, city, trail name, surface type, length, activity, and/or keywords regarding your interest. A number of listings include photos and reviews from people who've already visited the trail.

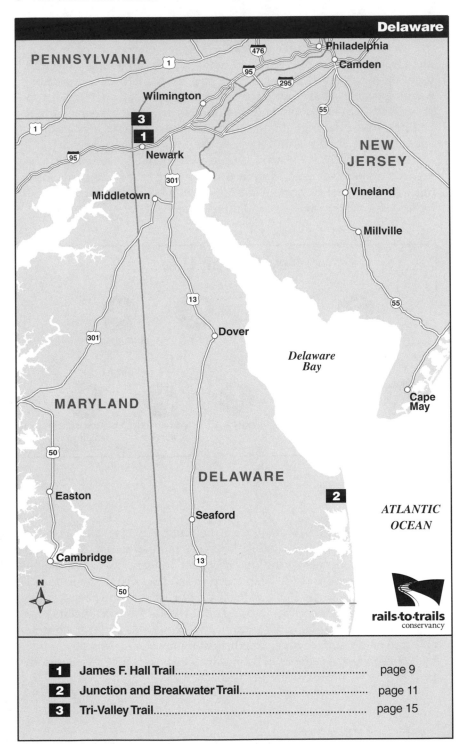

Delaware

PENNSYLVANIA

Philadelphia

Camden

Wilmington

3

1

Newark

Middletown

NEW JERSEY

Vineland

Millville

Dover

Delaware Bay

MARYLAND

Cape May

Easton

DELAWARE

2

ATLANTIC OCEAN

Seaford

Cambridge

N

rails·to·trails
conservancy

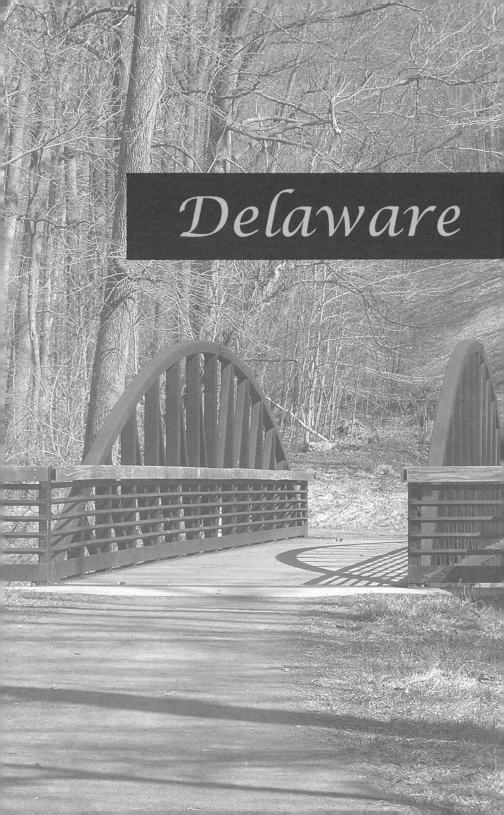

Delaware

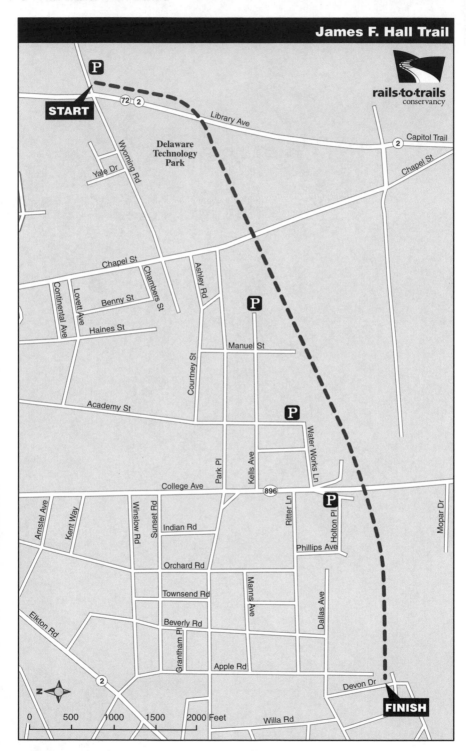

James F. Hall Trail

This rail-with-trail packs a lot into a short stretch: Its paved surface is great for bicycling, inline skating, and strolling, and there are multiple playgrounds, picnic areas, and access points along the route. Best of all, this urban trail never crosses a road, so you can coast uninterrupted for its entire length.

The trail also offers alternative transportation benefits, connecting Newark neighborhoods with a regional transit station, the University of Delaware, and shopping centers. If you're a train aficionado, it's almost guaranteed that you'll spot a car riding along the adjacent rail corridor, used by Amtrak, CSX, and the Southeastern Pennsylvania Transportation Authority (SEPTA). But you won't get too close to the trains, as a large fence separates the trail from the active rails.

Families with young children will especially enjoy this route, which passes three playgrounds featuring swings, slides, baseball diamonds, and soccer fields, plus basketball, handball, and tennis courts. The trail also crosses streams and wetlands and runs through a semi-forested area. Police call boxes are provided every tenth of a mile, and the trail is lit for use after dark.

Location
New Castle County

Endpoints
Delaware Technology Park at Wyoming Road to Bradford Lane

Mileage
1.7

Roughness Index
1

Surface
Asphalt

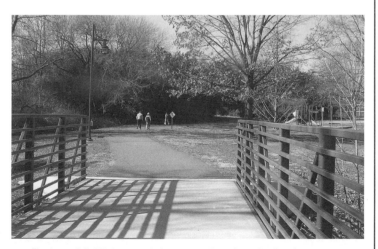

The James F. Hall Trail is a wonderful example of an urban rail-with-trail.

DIRECTIONS

To reach Delaware Technology Park at the northern end of the trail, from Interstate 95, take State Route 896 north toward downtown. Turn right on East Park Place, and then turn left onto South Chapel Street and right onto Wyoming Road. Park across from the College Square Shopping Center. The trail begins right at the intersection of Wyoming Road and Library Ave.

To reach College Ave./Septa Station, from Interstate 95, take State Route 896 (College Ave.) north to head downtown. After the University of Delaware field house and sports arena, go over an overpass. The trail is under this overpass. Take a quick left at the end of the overpass, where you will find parking and the Septa Station.

To reach Bradford Lane at the southeastern end of the trail, from Interstate 95, take State Route 896 north and turn left onto West Park Place. Turn left onto Apple Road, and then turn right onto Chrysler Ave. Turn right onto Bradford Lane, just after passing Devon Drive. The trail is at the end of the road. There is no dedicated parking at this location.

Contact: Newark Parks and Recreation
220 Elkton Road
Newark, DE 19711
(302) 366-7060
www.deldot.net/static/bike/hall_trail.html

This beautiful, pine-studded rail-trail winds through Cape Henlopen State Park next to wetlands and farmland, offering a break from the nearby beaches and eclectic shopping areas. The trail runs from Wolfe Neck in Lewes to the town of Rehoboth Beach and provides a perfect nature retreat.

The trail is mostly crushed stone, except for the last 0.2 mile near Rehoboth, when it becomes asphalt. As it is well-traveled by locals and tourists alike, be sure to remember your trail etiquette. You will be sharing the mostly flat route with bicyclists, walkers, runners, wheelchair users, and families with strollers and dogs.

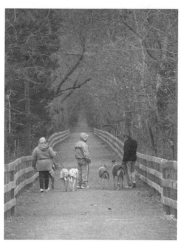

The Junction and Breakwater Trail is cool oasis in the pines in this Delaware beach town.

Pick up the trail at Wolfe Glade (off Wolfe Neck Road), a forested area of oak, hemlock, and pines. Turn left to head 0.6 mile to the trail's end, or turn right to head toward Rehoboth Beach. Along the way, the trail offers views of wetlands, especially at Holland Glade, via a refurbished 80-foot railroad bridge built in 1913. Continue farther and you'll find yourself flanked by cornfields and forests. Hawks, geese (both snow and Canada geese) can be spotted in the air, and deer, squirrels, and other small woodland animals share the trail.

At the trail's southern end, Tanger Outlets provides bargain hunters with an opportunity to break from the trail, shop the mall, and grab a bite to eat before heading back into the relative calm of the Junction and Breakwater Trail.

Location
Sussex County

Endpoints
Wolfe Neck to
Rehoboth Beach

Mileage
3

Roughness Index
1

Surface
Asphalt, ballast

Junction and Breakwater Trail

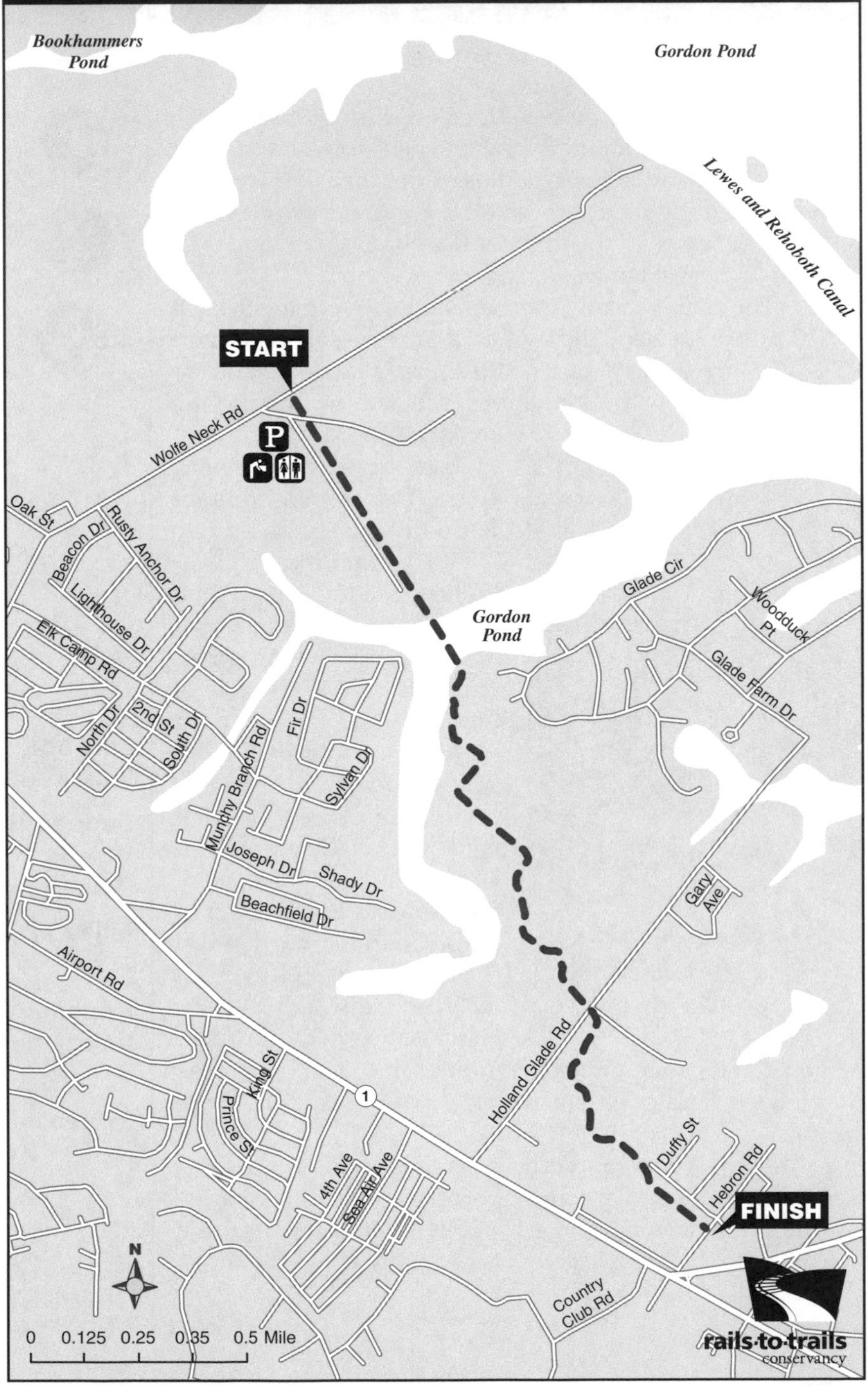

Bookhammers Pond

Gordon Pond

Lewes and Rehoboth Canal

START

Wolfe Neck Rd

P

Oak St

Beacon Dr

Rusty Anchor Dr

Lighthouse Dr

Elk Camp Rd

North Dr

2nd St

South Dr

Munphy Branch Rd

Fir Dr

Sylvan Dr

Joseph Dr

Shady Dr

Beachfield Dr

Airport Rd

King St

Prince St

4th Ave

Stag Ail Ave

Gordon Pond

Glade Cir

Woodduck Pt

Glade Farm Dr

Gacy Ave

Holland Glade Rd

Duffy St

Hebron Rd

FINISH

Country Club Rd

1

N

0   0.125 0.25   0.35   0.5 Mile

rails-to-trails
conservancy

DIRECTIONS

To reach Wolfe Neck, take State Route 1 to Lewes. If traveling north on Route 1, turn right onto Wolfe Neck Road. (If you are traveling south on Route 1, you will need to pass this turn and take a U-turn at the next traffic light in order to access Wolfe Neck Road. You can also go slightly farther south on Route 1 and turn left onto Munchy Branch Road, which you follow as it curves to the left until it hits Wolfe Neck Road.) You will see the Wolfe House on your right, where parking, restrooms, and a water fountain can be found next to the 0.2-mile path leading to the trail.

To reach the trail's end, from Rehoboth, take Route 1 toward the Tanger Outlets (36470 Seaside Outlet Drive in Rehoboth Beach). There is a bike/pedestrian path from the parking lot of the Tanger Outlets (look between the buildings in the middle) to the actual trail.

Contact: Delaware State Parks
89 Kings Hwy.
Dover, DE 19901
(302) 739-9220
www.destateparks.com/Activities/trails/J&B.htm

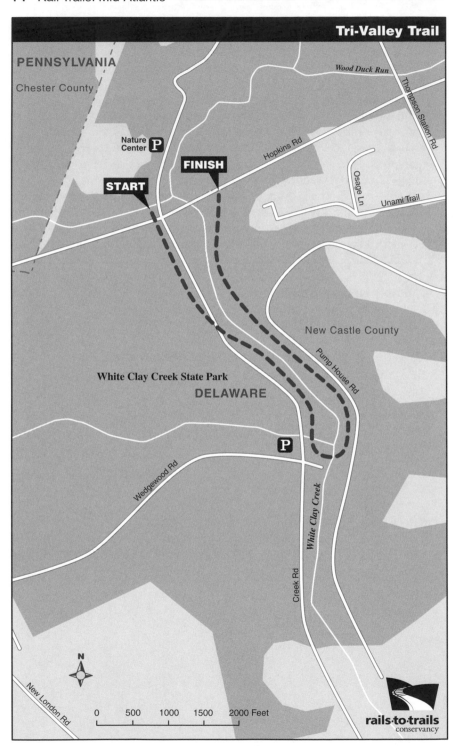

Tri-Valley Trail

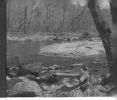

The Tri-Valley Trail is an easy-to-follow loop that begins and ends on Hopkins Road in White Clay Creek State Park near the park's nature center. The portion of the trail on the east side of White Clay Creek follows the path of the Pomeroy and Newark Railroad, which is why this trail is sometimes referred to as the Pomeroy Rail-Trail. The Pomeroy Railroad operated from 1873 to 1929, connecting Pomeroy, Pennsylvania, with Newark, Delaware, and Delaware City. The railroad was often referred to by locals as the "Pumpsie Doodle."

From the nature center parking lot, walk to Hopkins Road and cross it to find the beginning of the trail. After a mile, the trail turns left, passes the parking lot near Wedgewood Road, and then crosses a bridge over White Clay Creek. Most of this trail has a natural surface, but the trail developers put crushed stone down for a very short portion of the trail after the bridge. Follow the route of the crushed stone, as it is there to indicate the direction of this rail-trail. The old railroad was located on the side of the creek; look for a sign shortly after the bridge on your right that provides information on the railroad's history.

Location
New Castle County

Endpoints
White Clay Creek
State Park

Mileage
2

Roughness Index
2

Surface
Dirt

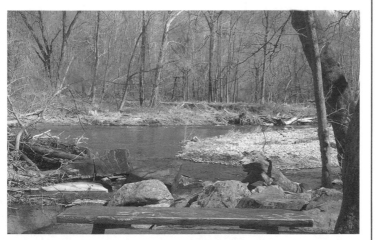

Loop trails are uncommon for most rail-trails, but this path gives you the best of both sides of White Clay Creek.

15

Along the way, the trail connects to several longer, steeper hiking/biking trails that cross the Mason-Dixon Line into Pennsylvania, but staying near the creek will keep you on the course of this rail-trail.

DIRECTIONS

To begin at the center of the trail, take State Route 896 (New London Road) northwest out of Newark. Turn right onto Wedgewood Road and follow it to the end. Parking is on the left, and the trail goes north and east of the parking lot.

Parking at the nature center can be reached by taking State Route 896 (New London Road) northwest of Newark. Turn right onto Hopkins Road after you pass the main entrance to White Clay Creek State Park, and follow the signs to the nature center. From there, backtrack on the road to the trail across Hopkins Road.

Contact: White Clay Creek State Park Nature Center
425 Wedgewood Road
Newark, DE 19711
(302) 368-6560
www.destateparks.com

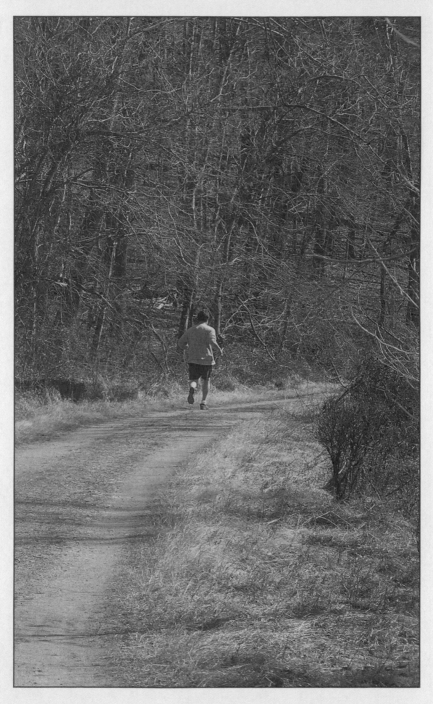

Tri-Valley Trail, Delaware

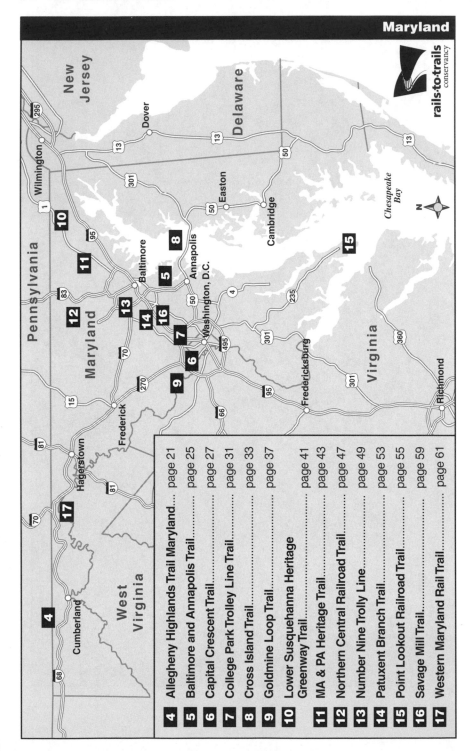

Maryland

rails•to•trails
conservancy

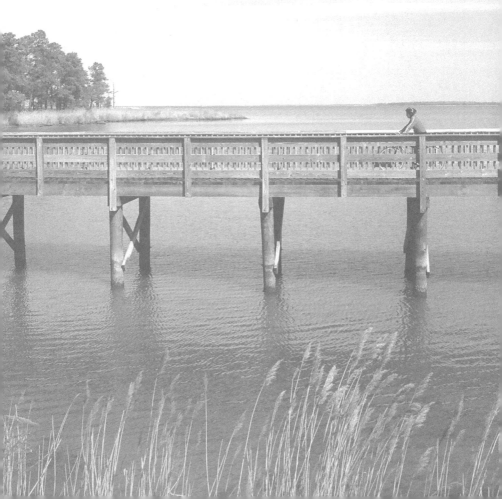

Maryland

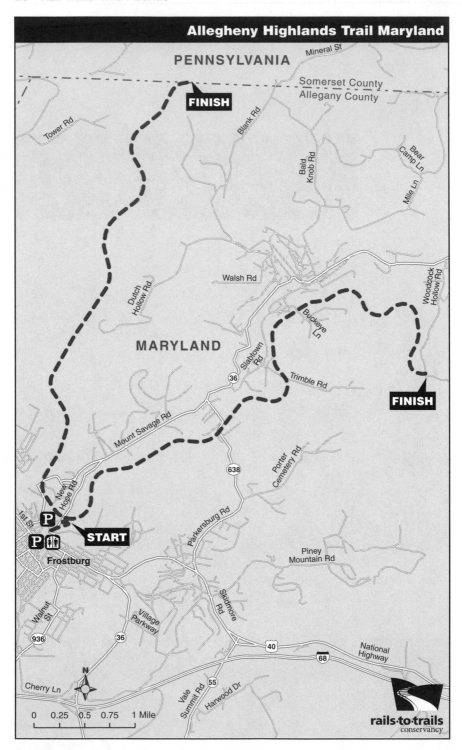

Allegheny Highlands Trail Maryland

PENNSYLVANIA

Mineral St

Somerset County
Allegany County

FINISH

Tower Rd

Blank Rd

Bald Knob Rd

Bear Camp Ln

Mile Ln

Dutch Hollow Rd

Walsh Rd

Woodcock Hollow Rd

MARYLAND

Buckeye Ln

Slabtown Rd

36

Trimble Rd

FINISH

Mount Savage Rd

638

Porter Cemetery Rd

New Hope Rd

1st St

P

P

START

Frostburg

Parkersburg Rd

Piney Mountain Rd

Walnut St

936

36

Village Parkway

Skidmore Rd

40

68

National Highway

Cherry Ln

N

0   0.25   0.5   0.75   1 Mile

Vale Summit Rd

55

Harwood Dr

rails·to·trails
conservancy

Allegheny Highlands Trail Maryland

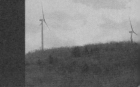

The Allegheny Highlands Trail Maryland (AHTM) follows the route of the historic Western Maryland Railroad for 11.5 miles from Woodcock Hollow Road to the Pennsylvania border. The AHTM parallels the Western Maryland Scenic Railroad and its operational steam locomotive, which provides scenic three-hour excursions to interested travelers.

The trail begins in the town of Frostburg at the Frostburg Depot, and from there heads in two directions—to Woodcock Hollow or the state boarder. The Frostburg Depot, constructed in 1891, served as a passenger and freight station. In 1989, the depot was restored as a restaurant, and it now serves as the endpoint of the Western Maryland Scenic Railroad tour.

Follow the AHTM north to travel toward the Mason-Dixon Line, which is approximately 5 miles from Frostburg. En route, you will pass through the Borden Tunnel, which was built in 1911 and is nearly 1000 feet long. On a hot day, it provides a refreshing release from the summer's heat. This relatively flat, crushed-limestone trail offers beautiful scenery of the rolling hills in

Location
Allegany County

Endpoints
Woodcock Hollow Road to Maryland-Pennsylvania State Line

Mileage
11.5

Roughness Index
2

Surface
Crushed stone, asphalt

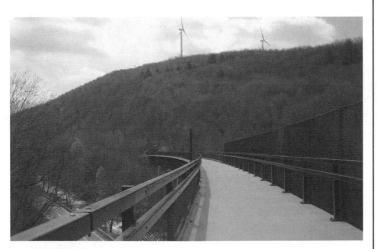

The long bridge span on the Allegheny Highlands Trail Maryland offers a view from the old railroad's perspective.

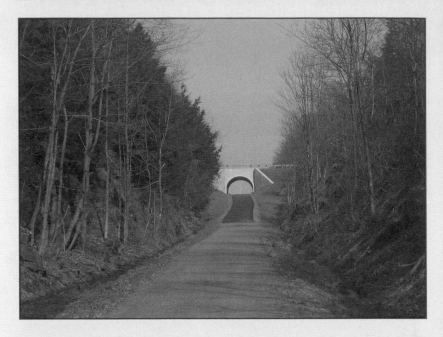

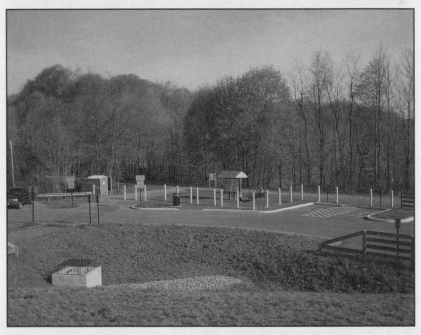

Top: Tunnels beneath roadways are often constructed to provide rail-trail users with safe, traffic-free passage.
Below: Trailheads often offer amenities such as drinking fountains, restrooms, parking, bike racks, and maps.

western Maryland. The Mason-Dixon Line rests at the state border between Maryland and Pennsylvania and is the official end of the AHTM. However, the trail continues as the Great Allegheny Passage all the way to Pittsburgh.

The AHTM also travels approximately 6 miles east from Frostburg to Woodcock Hollow Road. This section of the trail also follows the historic Western Maryland Scenic Railroad. At the time of this writing, construction was underway to finish the remaining 9-mile section of the trail connecting it with Cumberland. When complete, the entire trail will be more than 20 miles long and will connect to the nearly 1000-foot-long Brush Tunnel, also built in 1911. The tunnel will also be shared with the Western Maryland Scenic Railroad.

DIRECTIONS

From Cumberland, take Interstate 68 west and exit at MD Route 36 (exit 34) to head north toward Frostburg. Turn left onto Main Street (US Route 40). In less than a mile, turn right onto Depot Road, just past the Domino's Pizza. Follow Depot Road to the Old Depot Train Station. Turn right onto New Hope Road and follow it for less than a quarter mile. Trailhead parking is located on the right.

To reach the trailhead at Woodcock Hollow Road, follow MD Route 36 north from Frostburg to Barrellville, and turn right onto Woodcock Hollow Road. The trailhead is approximately a mile down Woodcock Hollow Road on the right.

Contact: Allegheny Highlands Trail Maryland
PO Box 28
Cumberland, MD 21501
(301) 687-4428
www.ahtmtrail.org

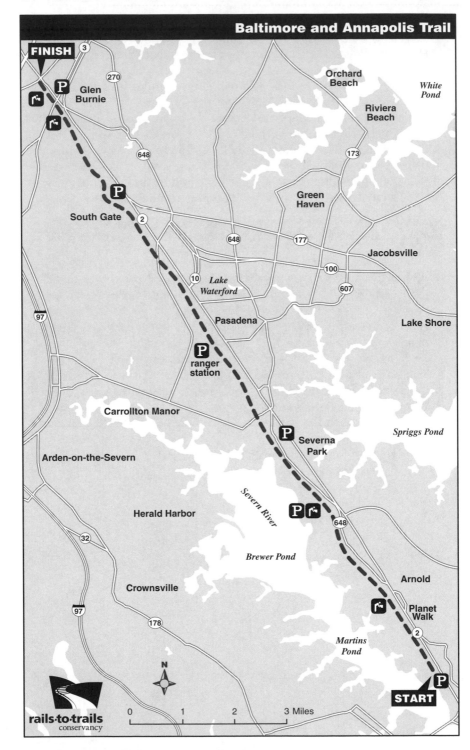

Baltimore and Annapolis Trail

FINISH

Glen Burnie

Orchard Beach

White Pond

Riviera Beach

South Gate

Green Haven

Jacobsville

Lake Waterford

Pasadena

Lake Shore

ranger station

Carrollton Manor

Spriggs Pond

Arden-on-the-Severn

Severna Park

Severn River

Herald Harbor

Brewer Pond

Arnold

Crownsville

Planet Walk

Martins Pond

N

START

rails·to·trails
conservancy

0   1   2   3 Miles

Baltimore and Annapolis Trail

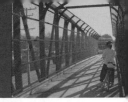

If you are looking to augment your physical workout with some intellectual exercise, try out the Baltimore and Annapolis Trail, or the B&A Trail. This scenic, paved path is more than just a trail—it's a history lesson and tour through our solar system.

The trail follows the route of the Annapolis and Baltimore Short Line, which started running freight and passenger service in 1880 and helped shape this suburban region near the nation's capital. Today, the trail is a 112-acre linear park that winds through parks, neighborhoods, and natural wooded areas. The trail also passes the Marley Station shopping mall, and the ranger station at mile marker 6.3, where public grills and a large field make an ideal picnic stop. Portions of the trail are sponsored by trail volunteers who tend the flowerbeds and kiosks along the trail.

Along the trail, you will find a literal alphabet of historical markers, from A to Z. The A marker, at mile 0.1, is the Winchester Station House at Manresa, near the Annapolis start of the trail. At mile 13.3, you will find the Z marker identifying the Sawmill Branch, the area's source of water and power in the early 18th cen-

Location
Howard and Anne Arundel counties

Endpoints
Annapolis (Jonas Green Park) to Glen Burnie (Dorsey Road)

Mileage
13.3

Roughness Index
1

Surface
Asphalt

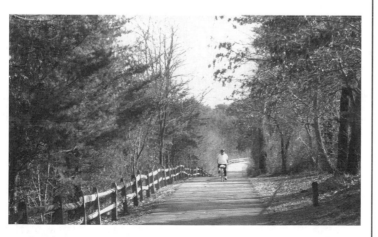

The Baltimore and Annapolis Trail is one for all seasons—from stunning leaf color in the fall to blooming trailside gardens in the spring.

tury. To follow along with each marker, pick up a flyer at the ranger station.

Near Harundale Mall at mile 12, you will come upon the Planet Walk, a linear museum with educational displays for the sun and each planet. Sponsored by NASA, the planets are true to scale and each has an educational storyboard about our solar system.

The trail, and its educational opportunities, end in the small town of Glen Burnie. But you may continue on the BWI Trail loop that connects to the north end of the trail for an additional 12.5 miles around the Baltimore Washington International Airport.

DIRECTIONS

The Annapolis trailhead is located off US Route 50 past the Severn River. Take exit 27 and head south toward the Naval Academy on MD Route 450. The parking lot for Jonas Green Park is on the right. There are directions to the trail on the board near the entrance of the parking lot.

To reach the Glen Burnie trailhead, take US Route 50 east from Washington, DC, to exit 21 and follow Interstate 97 north. Take exit 15 leading to MD Route 176 west (Dorsey Road). Continue on 176 before turning right onto MD Route 648 (Baltimore and Annapolis Blvd.). At the first light, take a right on Crain Hwy. and then take a right onto Central Ave. The parking lot is on the right and runs along the trail.

Contact: Maryland Department of Natural Resources
580 Taylor Ave, E2
Annapolis MD 21401
(410) 260-8778
www.dnr.state.md.us/greenways/b&a_trail.html

Capital Crescent Trail

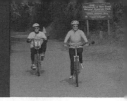

The 11-mile Capital Crescent Trail follows the route of the Baltimore and Ohio Railroad's Georgetown Branch rail line of the Baltimore and Ohio Railroad. It begins in downtown Silver Spring east of the Rock Creek Trestle and curves westward and south through Maryland and into Washington, DC, to end in the heart of historic Georgetown. Someday, the section between downtown Silver Spring and Bethesda, Maryland, will be paved and officially become part of the Capital Crescent, but until then this section is actually called the Georgetown Branch Trail.

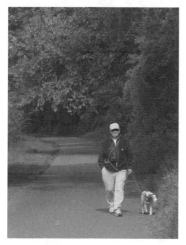

A thick canopy of trees shades parts of the Capital Crescent Trail.

The asphalt section of the trail connects Georgetown to Bethesda. In Georgetown, the trail travels with the Potomac River on one side and the Chesapeake & Ohio Canal National Historical Park towpath on the other side. From the trail, you can watch the rowing crews of Georgetown University at practice or possibly jog past a senator. Deer, foxes, rabbits, many species of birds, and, of course, the three colors of ubiquitous Washington, DC, squirrels—white, grey, and black—also share the trail.

In Georgetown near Thompsons Boat Center and in west Silver Spring at Jones Mill Road, the trail connects to Rock Creek Park, a densely forested area that closes its roads to car traffic on the weekend and becomes a playground for non-motorized uses. The loop of the Capital Crescent and Rock Creek Park totals 22 miles and takes you past the National Zoological Park and the Kennedy Center.

Location
Montgomery County, Maryland, and Washington, DC

Endpoints
Silver Spring, Maryland, to Georgetown in Washington, DC

Mileage
11

Roughness Index
1

Surface
Asphalt, crushed stone, gravel

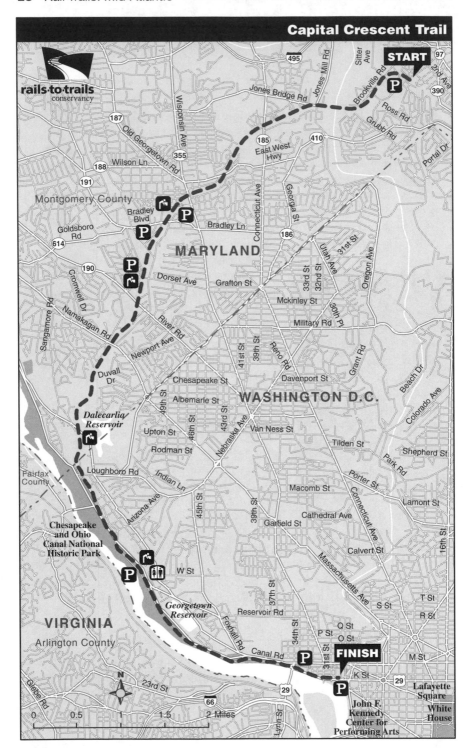

In Silver Spring, Bethesda, and Georgetown, there are a number of places just off the trail to have a meal or a cup of coffee, as well as a large number of shops.

DIRECTIONS

To reach the Silver Spring terminus from Washington's Capital Beltway (Interstate 495), take the Georgia Ave. exit and head south toward Silver Spring. Turn right on Colesville Road toward the Metro station. At the first light, turn right onto Second Ave. The Georgetown Branch Trail starts at this intersection.

To start in Bethesda, take the Capital Beltway to the MD Route 355 (Wisconsin Ave.) exit and head south toward Bethesda. In downtown Bethesda, turn right onto Bethesda Ave. The trail crosses Bethesda Ave. at Woodmont Ave., just one block west of Wisconsin Ave.

To begin in the Georgetown neighborhood of Washington, DC, go south on Wisconsin Ave. to its end under the Whitehurst Freeway and turn right onto Water Street. The trail begins at the end of Water Street. Street parking is usually available along Water Street on weekends.

Contact: Coalition for the Capital Crescent Trail
PO Box 30703
Bethesda, MD 20824
(202) 234-4874
www.cctrail.org

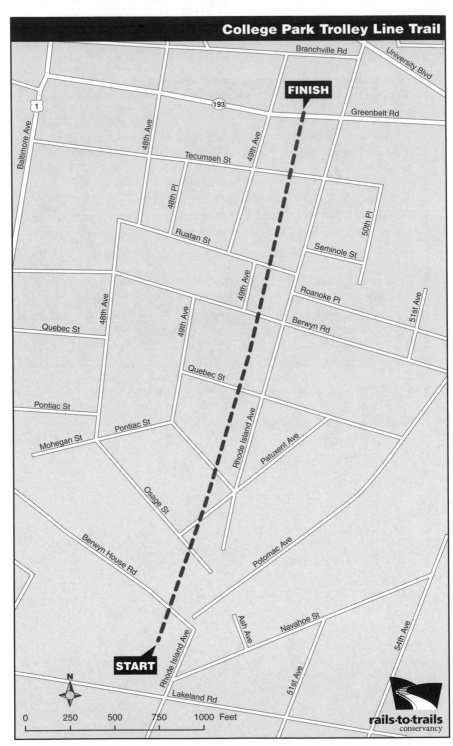

College Park Trolley Line Trail

College Park Trolley Line Trail

The College Park Trolley Line Trail provides a safe pathway for students, from kindergartners to doctoral candidates, to walk and bike to school in College Park. The short, paved trail follows the route of the trolley that once ran from Washington, DC, to Laurel between 1903 and the mid-'50s. With service roads on either side of the trail, trail users have easy access to three schools, and there is a partial route for college students heading to nearby University of Maryland.

Of course, you don't have to be earning a degree to use the trail. Local residents use the path for after-dinner walks, commuters take it as a shortcut to the Metrorail system, and house cats find it a good place to wait for an indulgent hand to give them a pat. The trail sits on a raised berm and crosses several quiet neighborhood roads, where you can easily pick up the pathway. Plans for expansion of the trail will enable the pathway to connect to a series of long trails around the region, and link all of College Park, end to end.

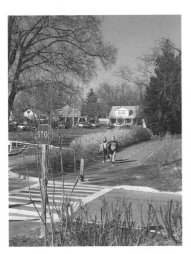

In this university town, the College Park Trolley Line Trail brings together people of all ages.

Mostly shaded nearly all year by walnut, maple, and flowering trees that tower near the trail from neighboring yards, the rail-trail also serves as something of a home-and-garden tour. Residents of the quirky Sears bungalows and rambling colonials along the trail use their yards to showcase their green thumbs. Additionally, several businesses within a block of trail, including an impressive herb shop and a corner convenience store, provide diversions during a short stroll.

Location
Prince George's County

Endpoints
Berwyn House Road to Greenbelt Road

Mileage
0.6

Roughness Index
1

Surface
Asphalt

DIRECTIONS

To get to the start point from Washington's beltway, Interstate 495, take exit 25B south on MD Route 1. Turn right onto Berwyn House Road and look for the trailhead on the right in two blocks. Parking is on the street.

Contact: College Park Area Bicycle Coalition
5206 Paducah Road
College Park, MD 20740
www.cpabc.org/home.htm

Cross Island Trail

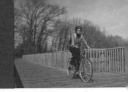

Maryland's Cross Island Trail spans Kent Island in Queen Anne's County, providing multiple points of access to everything from libraries and schools, to ball fields and the waterfront. It's an impressively signed, well-maintained, beautiful community asset.

Begin at Terrapin Nature Park, a parcel of protected land for birds and native plant life. Just past the nature area, to the left of the trail, is an old graveyard with less than a dozen cracked and weather headstones tucked into the trees. If you can spot it, it's worth a peak. From here, the trail quickly winds through light residential neighborhoods and stands of white pines and hemlocks.

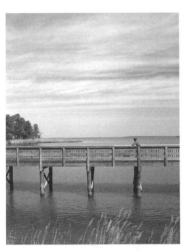

The Cross Island Trail skirts inlets of the Chesapeake Bay.

At the first mile marker, you come to Old Love Point Park, a recreation area with baseball and soccer fields. Continuing along, the trail passes through farm fields, and you'll be able to see a lighthouse in the distance that indicates how close you really are to the seashore.

At mile 3.8, you will have to do a short, back-road jog to reconnect with the trail, but a blue-painted bike lane makes this a simple transition. Back on the path, you'll come to a long wooden bridge that provides the first unhindered view of the water. This lovely expanse is a gem of the Cross Island Trail.

Before reaching the marina in Kent Narrows, you must head uphill to cross over the causeway on the parallel US Hwy. 50, where there is an extremely wide shoulder. At the marina, you have a choice: Head to the

Location
Queen Anne's County

Endpoints
Terrapin Nature Park to Kent Narrows, Kent Island

Mileage
5.5

Roughness Index
1

Surface
Asphalt

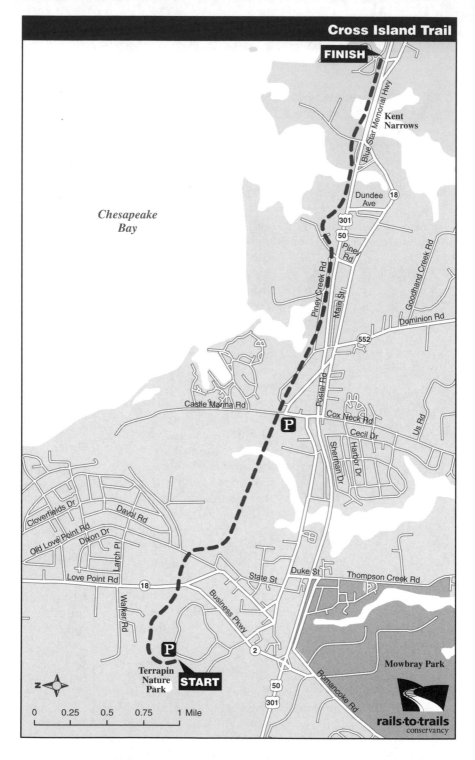

left to Chesapeake Exploration Center, or head the right to continue along the trail. Here, the trail becomes a series of sidewalks and access points to the waterfront and its restaurants and boat slips.

DIRECTIONS

To reach the start at Terrapin Nature Park, from Annapolis, take US Hwy. 50 east to exit 37 (the first exit after crossing the Chesapeake Bay Bridge) and turn left onto MD Route 8. Follow Route 8 to the second light and turn left into Chesapeake Bay Business Park. Follow the road to the right around the circle until you come to Terrapin Nature Park. There is ample parking and portable toilets are at the trailhead.

To reach Kent Narrows, take US Hwy. 50 east from Annapolis. After crossing the Bay Bridge, travel across Kent Island. Cross the Narrows on a bridge and turn left onto MD Route 835 (Kent Narrows Road). Parking is to the left under the bridge.

Contact: Queen Anne's County
Department of Parks and Recreation
1945 4-H Park Road
Centreville, MD 21617
(410) 758-0835
www.qac.org

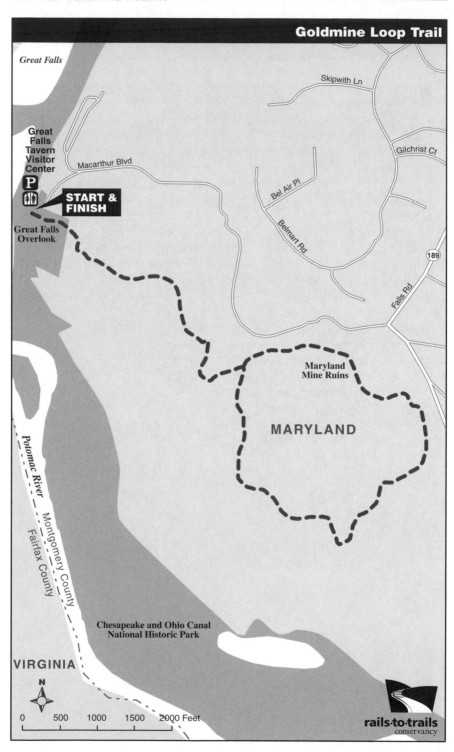

Goldmine Loop Trail

Great Falls

Skipwith Ln

Great Falls Tavern Visitor Center

Gilchrist Ct

Macarthur Blvd

Bel Air Pl

START & FINISH

Belmart Rd

Great Falls Overlook

189

Falls Rd

Maryland Mine Ruins

MARYLAND

Potomac River

Montgomery County
Fairfax County

Chesapeake and Ohio Canal National Historic Park

VIRGINIA

N

0   500   1000   1500   2000 Feet

rails·to·trails
conservancy

Goldmine Loop Trail

Tucked in the meandering, wooded hills of the sprawling yet understated multimillion-dollar estates of Great Falls, just outside Washington, DC, is the Chesapeake & Ohio Canal National Historic Park. Home to the already famous C&O Canal Towpath, the Great Falls section of the park also hosts this unique rail-trail circuit.

The trail begins at the hillside just beyond the historic, early 1800s-era Great Falls Tavern Visitor Center. Start at the well-marked post and head up a series of stairs that are cut into the hillside and reinforced with logs. This is not your traditional rail-trail. Only part of it runs on the former railroad corridor, so prepare for some gentle uphill climbs. (The trail is off-limits to bicycles.)

The trail, marked by a blue blaze, immediately takes you into the surrounding airy forest. After less than a mile, you reach the beginning of the actual loop. Take note: Detours on yellow-blazed spur trails along the route take you to the Maryland Mine ruins, where gold was processed from 1867 to 1939.

Upon reaching the start of the loop, go either left or right; both ways will take you back to this starting

Location
Montgomery County

Endpoints
Great Falls Tavern Visitor Center

Mileage
3.2

Roughness Index
1

Surface
Asphalt

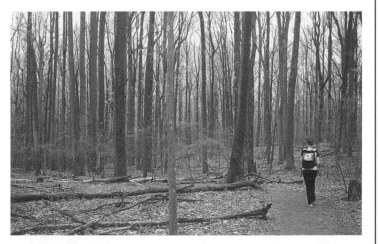

When you're in the woods here, it's hard to imagine that the marble halls of Washington, DC, are only 20 miles away.

point. If you head to the right, you will first come to the Woodland Trail Spur (one of six trail spurs along the loop), where you'll cross a tiny creek and the surface will change from dirt to gravel. If you are on the trail in the spring, several stands of red bud will be in bloom, providing a vibrant color contrasts to the grayish-green of an awakening forest. At certain points, you may have to scramble over, under, or around impressive, felled trees, but they only add to the trail's woodland feel.

When you return to the beginning of the loop, take the path back down to the visitor center and explore the rest of the park. Don't miss the nearby Great Falls overlook, which provides stunning views of the waterfall that separates the upper from the lower Potomac River. Pick up a trail map at the ranger station to find directions to the overlook.

DIRECTIONS

From the Washington, DC's beltway–Interstate 495–take exit 41 (Carderock/Great Falls) to follow the Clara Barton Parkway. At the stop sign at the end of road, turn left onto Macarthur Blvd. Go 3.5 miles to the end of the road at the park. Entry is $5 per car, and there is ample parking.

Contact: Great Falls Tavern Visitor Center
11710 MacArthur Blvd.
Potomac, MD 20854
(301) 767-3714
www.nps.gov/archive/choh/Visitor/Centers/
GreatFalls.html

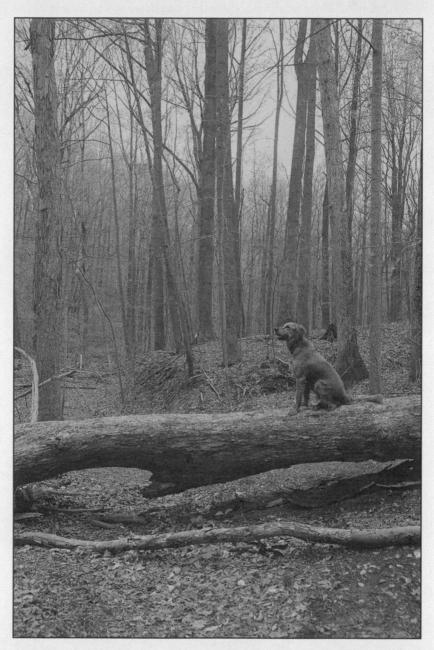

A felled tree across the path doesn't stop the more adventurous trail users on the Goldmine Loop Trail.

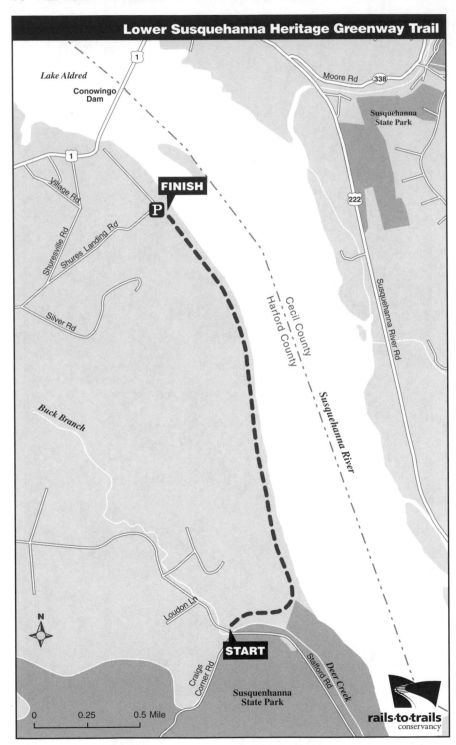

Lower Susquehanna Heritage Greenway Trail

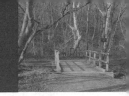

Maryland's Susquehanna State Park is recognized for challenging hiking and biking trails, camping facilities, rock outcroppings, boating, a museum, and restored historical sites. But none of these outshines the Susquehanna River, which sweeps majestically by, beckoning fishermen and nature lovers.

One way to take in the scenic river is by venturing out on the rail-trail along its western bank. The Philadelphia Electric Company built the corridor in 1926 to transport materials from Havre d'Grace on the Chesapeake Bay to the construction site of the new Conowingo Dam. The dam was completed in two years and the rail line, no longer needed, became a victim of overgrowth and erosion until the Lower Susquehanna Heritage Greenway Trail was created. Eventually, it will extend 50 miles along both sides on the river; presently, only 2.5 miles are open.

To start the trail from the south, in Susquehanna State Park, go to north side of the Deer Creek bridge. Near this end, where the trail travels inland to the sparkling Deer Creek, is the site of the early Stafford flint furnace, with a portion of the furnace still standing.

Location
Cecil and Harford counties

Endpoints
Susquehanna State Park to Conowingo Dam

Mileage
2.5

Roughness Index
1

Surface
Crushed stone

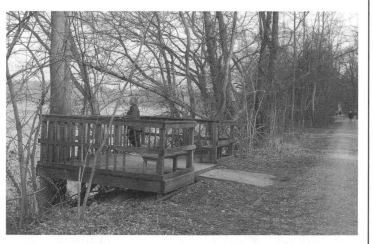

Views of the Susquehanna River prompt trail users to take a break from their trip.

Along the way to the impressive 4648-foot-long, 102-foot-high Conowingo Dam, you'll pass wooded wetlands harboring songbirds and abundant wildflowers, especially in the spring. You may also spot old rail tracks and informational displays with historical and scientific details about the area.

The wide, stone-dust trail is easy to walk or bike, and although there is a dense canopy overhead offering shade in the summer months, the river views are frequent and beautiful. Near the northern end, a viewing platform provides river access to anglers, bird-watchers (the dam is a feeding ground for many varieties), and the curious.

DIRECTIONS

To start from the south, follow MD Route 155 north from Interstate 95 and turn right on Lapidum Road. Take a left on Stafford Road and follow it to Susquehanna State Park and the Deer Creek picnic area on the north end.

To reach the northern trailhead, take Interstate 95 north from Baltimore to exit 85. Follow MD Route 22 north to MD Route 136, continuing north. Upon reaching US Route 1, go north. Turn right on Shuresville Road and then left on Shures Landing Road. Follow this to Conowingo Dam and look for the trailhead just south of the dam at Fisherman's Park.

Contact: Lower Susquehanna Heritage Greenway, Inc.
4948 Conowingo Road
Conowingo, MD 21034
(410) 457-2482
www.lshgreenway.org

MA & PA Heritage Trail

In the early 1900s, the Maryland and Pennsylvania Railroad screamed through the Harford County countryside, heralding industrial progress. Today, a new kind of progress is evident in the sound of twittering birds and babbling brooks on the long-deserted rail line. This refreshing natural oasis found on the MA & PA Heritage Trail lures visitors and residents of the neighborhoods just steps from the path.

The trail is in two sections, with nearly 2 miles between them. If you plan to travel both portions, use a map to determine the best on-road route between the two segments. Both segments have ample parking and are easy to navigate, with a surface of stone dust and some paving on slopes in the town of Bel Air.

The 2-mile southern section, in Bel Air, weaves through old stands of native trees, rising and falling with the dips of the landscape. It travels past streams and over bridges, and though homes are visible at the far reaches of the trees, this lovely green space provides a protected natural environment and a perfect setting for a stroll or a short jog.

Location
Harford County

Endpoints
Bel Air to Forest Hill

Mileage
3.5

Roughness Index
1

Surface
Crushed stone, dirt

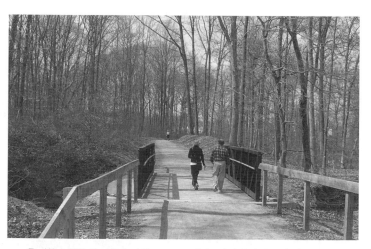

The MA & PA Heritage Trail, which cuts a wooded path through this suburban area, takes its names from the Maryland (MA) and Pennsylvania (PA) Railroad.

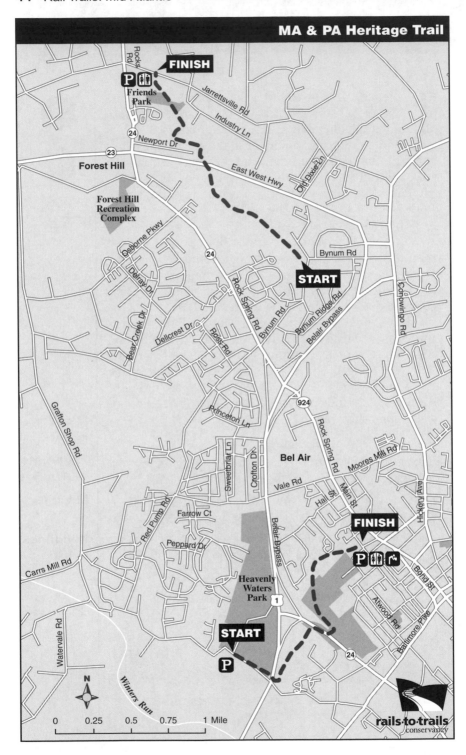

MA & PA Heritage Trail

In Forest Hill, the rail-trail meanders for 1.5 miles past an enchanting marsh teeming with wildlife, and through tidy developments of suburban homes, a light industrial area, and a recreational field.

North or south, the community parks framing the endpoints of the MA & PA Heritage Trail beckon you to slow down, enjoy a picnic, or watch the sun go down.

DIRECTIONS

To access the Bel Air segment, follow Interstate 95 to exit 77B and take MD Route 24 (Vietnam Vets Memorial Hwy.) north toward Bel Air. Turn left onto Baltimore Pike. Turn right on North Tollgate Road and go 1 mile. The trail endpoint is on the right; parking is available here, across the road, and also at the Williams Street endpoint in Bel Air.

To access the Forest Hill segment, take MD Route 24 north from Bel Air to East West Hwy. (State Route 23), and turn left. Drive for about 2 miles, and turn right on Rock Spring Road (State Route 24). Follow this for about a half mile and turn left onto East Jarrettville Road. In a quarter mile, look for Friends Park on the left. Turn left into the park and follow the drive past the pond and up the rise to the trailhead, or meet the trail at Melrose Lane off Bynum Road.

Contact: Harford County Parks and Recreation
702 N. Tollgate Road
Bel Air, MD 21014
(410) 638-3572
www.harfordcountymd.gov/parks%5Frec/
ma_pa_corridor.htm

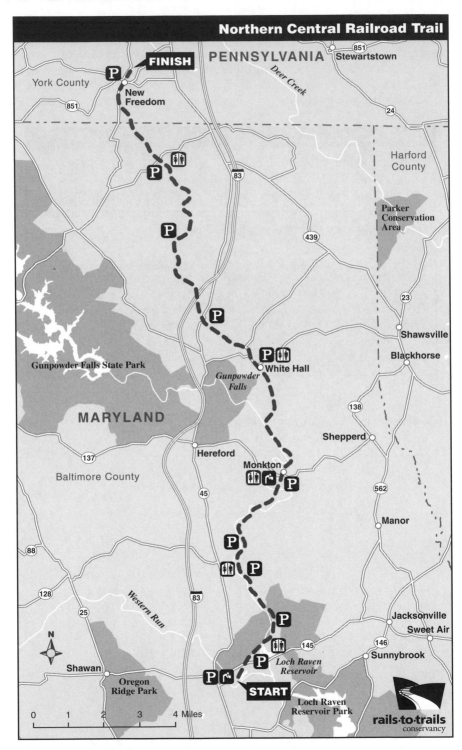

Northern Central Railroad Trail

The Northern Central Railroad Trail, completed in 1984, is one of the best hiking and biking trails in the Mid-Atlantic region. It allows for more than 20 miles of smooth, flat travel on the crushed stone surface, punctuated by a number of access points and an abundance of trees that provide refreshing shade on hot summer days. The trail begins in Cockeysville, Maryland, a suburb of Baltimore, and ends just over the state line in New Freedom, Pennsylvania, where the Mason-Dixon Line divides the southern Atlantic states from the Northeastern states.

The history of the rail-trail dates back to 1832, when the Northern Central Railroad carried passengers, people vacationing at Bentley Springs, and freight between Baltimore and York or Harrisburg, Pennsylvania. The railroad ran for about 140 years, and you can still see part of the old bed, which was converted to a rail-tail in the early 1980s. Today, the Northern Central Railroad Trail is managed by the Maryland Department of Natural Resources as part of the Gunpowder Falls State Park.

Amenities along the route include picnic and park benches, drinking fountains for hikers and bikers and

Location
Baltimore County

Endpoints
Cockeysville, Maryland, to New Freedom, Pennsylvania

Mileage
22

Roughness Index
1

Surface
Crushed stone

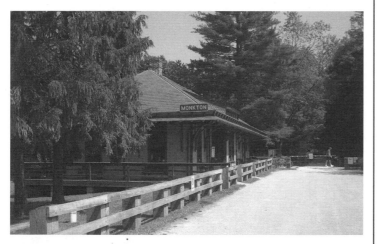

A restored train depot in Monkton is now the Northern Central Railroad Trail's information center.

47

dogs, too, and portable restrooms. Just off the trail, you can enjoy a small art gallery, an antique shop, and several places to stop and buy food and drinks. Hotels and motels can be found within a mile of the trail, and there is easy access to a bike shop that rents and repairs bikes. The trail cuts through several charming towns, including Monkton (a major stop for hikers and bikers), Parkton, Falls Overlook, Bentley Springs, and New Freedom.

The trail is used by an eclectic mix of horseback riders, joggers, walkers, hikers, bikers, and people of all ages. On the weekends, the trail is heavily used by local residents and travelers from the Baltimore area, so parking may be a challenge. For those seeking an escape from the urban areas of the Mid-Atlantic and Northeast region, this trail is a wooded oasis—an escape from the every day stresses of nearby city life.

DIRECTIONS

To reach the southern end of the trail from the neighborhood of Ashland, follow Interstate 83 north from Baltimore, and take exit 20 to Cockeysville. Turn left on York Road (MD Route 45), and then turn right on Ashland Road, which is a T-intersection. Ashland turns into Paper Mill Road. The trail parking lot will be on the left.

Contact: Gunpowder Falls State Park
PO Box 480
2813 Jerusalem Road
Kingsville, MD 21087
(410) 592-2897
www.dnr.state.md.us/publiclands/central/
gunpowder.html

Number Nine Trolly Line

The first thing you may notice about Number Nine Trolly Line (also known as Trolly Line #9) is the boardwalk that curves between the canyons of massive rock. The granite was hand-cut in the 1890s when the electric streetcar rails were built from Ellicott City to Catonsville, and today, these 100-foot walls are a striking gateway to the trail from historic Ellicott City just across the Patapsco River from Oella.

The boardwalk quickly gives way to pavement as the trail winds uphill through the woods. On your left,

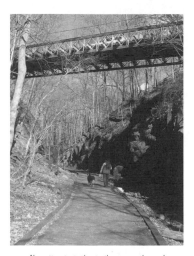

Near its start, the trail passes through a cut in the rock on a boardwalk, beneath an automobile bridge.

a babbling stream feeding into the Patapsco River provides a peaceful soundtrack to your journey. Tall shade trees keep the trail—and you—cool as you climb through woodlands and occasionally pass homes that border the trail. Near the 1-mile mark, a short detour off the trail will take you to Banneker Historical Park & Museum, which has nature trails, archaeological sites, and living history areas re-creating the colonial farm and life of Benjamin Banneker, an African-American astronomer and farmer.

Back on the trail, the rustic scenery gives way to a more suburban landscape. The few road crossings are well-marked and the gradual slope makes for a pleasant trip both up- and downhill. When you reach the end of the trail, simply turn around and head back downhill to enjoy Ellicott City, including the Baltimore & Ohio Train Museum, which highlights the history of the nation's first railroad.

Location
Baltimore County

Endpoints
Oella to Catonsville

Mileage
1.5

Roughness Index
1

Surface
Asphalt

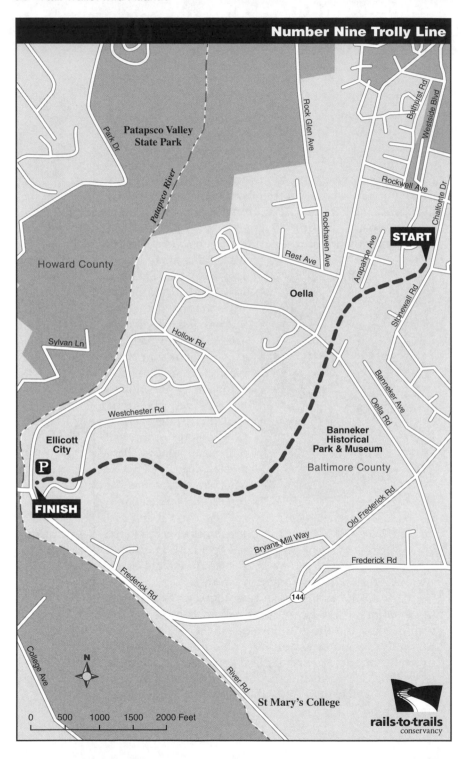

DIRECTIONS

To get to Oella from downtown Ellicott City, take MD Route 144 (Frederick Road) east to the Patapsco River, where the road becomes Main Street. Cross the river and take an immediate left (north) onto Oella Road, where you will find trail parking on your right (the river is on your left). You must climb stairs to get to the trail from here.

To get to Catonsville from downtown Ellicott City, follow MD Route 144 (Frederick Road) east past the Patapsco River and turn north (left) onto Westchester Ave., where you will find parking that is accessible to disabled users.

Contact: Maryland Greenways Commission
580 Taylor Ave., E2
Annaplois, MD 21401
(410) 260-8778
www.dnr.state.md.us/greenways/
counties/baltimore.html

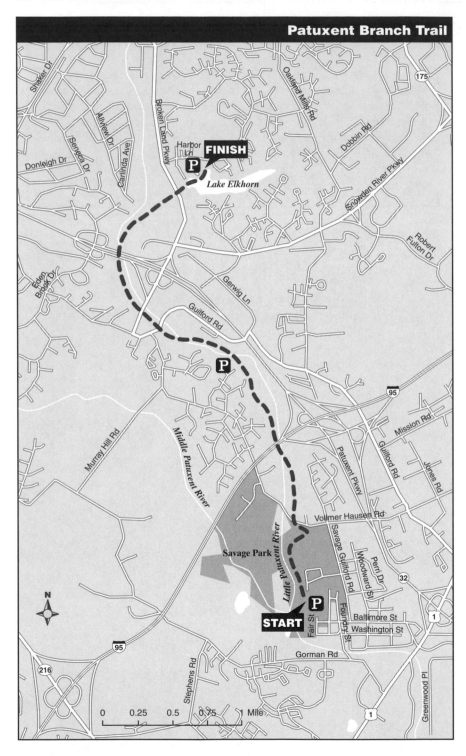

Patuxent Branch Trail

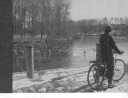

The Patuxent Branch Trail is part of a 20-mile trail system over and around the rolling hills of Howard County that follows a former Baltimore and Ohio Railroad line along the Patuxent River.

The trail begins in Savage Park. Follow signs along the trail indicating the direction to Lake Elkhorn. When you reach Vollmer Hausen Road, turn left and stay on the sidewalk to find the trail where it picks up on the other side of the road at the bottom of this short hill. A crosswalk eases you across this busy road.

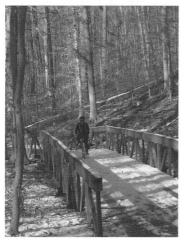

Bridges along the trail make the going easier on this mixed-surface trail in Savage Park.

A little more than half of the trail is paved, and the other half has a gravel surface. A small portion of the trail includes a bridle path. Ten bridges help keep you dry as you travel through this flood plain. The most impressive, the 1902 Guilford Pratt Truss Bridge, is a symbol of Howard County's two most important industries—the railroad and the granite quarry. Signs along the trail explain the historical significance of both industries, and the trail will take you straight through the grounds of a quarry that operated until 1928.

The rail-trail ends at Lake Elkhorn, but picnic facilities, a playground, parking, a boat slip, and a walking and biking path around the lake may keep you going. Or you can head back to the Savage Park entrance of the Patuxent Branch Trail and pick up the flatter and shorter Savage Mill Trail (see page 59) that begins just a few blocks away.

Location
Howard County

Endpoints
Savage (Savage Park) to Columbia (Lake Elkhorn)

Mileage
4.5

Roughness Index
1

Surface
Asphalt, crushed stone, concrete

53

DIRECTIONS

To access the Savage Park entrance from Interstate 95, take MD Route 32 (Patuxent Parkway) east, and then turn right on US Route 1 (Baltimore Washington Blvd.), heading south toward Laurel. Turn right on Gorman Road, and then turn right on Foundry Street. Turn left onto Washington Street and follow it to the end, where you take a right onto Fair Street, which ends at the park. Take the road in the parking lot to the right until it ends at a smaller parking lot at the trailhead.

To access the Lake Elkhorn entrance from Interstate 95, take MD Route 32 (Patuxent Parkway) west and then take the Broken Land Parkway north toward Owen Brown. The lake (and a parking lot next to the playground and boat slip) will be on your right.

Contact: Howard County Recreation and Parks Department
7120 Oakland Mills Road
Columbia, MD 21046
(410) 313-4687
www.co.ho.md.us/RAP/RAP_HomePage.htm

Point Lookout Railroad Trail

The Point Lookout Railroad Trail (also called Periwinkle Point Nature Trail) follows a corridor that was cleared in the early 1800s for a planned railroad line connecting Point Lookout, Maryland, to Washington, DC. Active rail service came to some portions of the corridor over the years, but this 1-mile section was never completed. Today it is still quiet, as a peaceful dirt path running through historic Point Lookout State Park.

The trail entrance is located near the southern end of the trail. Here you will find the Civil War Museum/Marshland Nature Center, where you can stop in from May to September to learn more about the park's history as a Civil War prison camp.

From the start, bear right for a leisurely walk on the trail's northern—and longer—section. The trail is bordered by 6-foot-high reeds and pine trees and provides an occasional glimpse of the Point Lookout Creek. Marshy areas are found immediately adjacent to the trail and occasionally the trail itself is waterlogged, requiring slight off-trail navigation. This section of the trail ends in an open, privately owned field.

Location
St. Mary's County

Endpoints
Point Lookout State Park

Mileage
1

Roughness Index
2

Surface
Dirt, grass

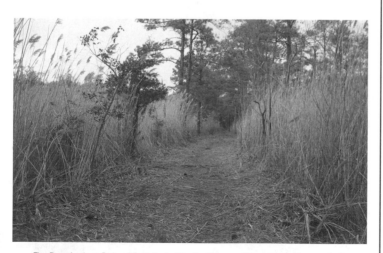

The Point Lookout Railroad Trail, flanked by the Potomac River and the Chesapeake Bay, is an excellent place to spot waterfowl.

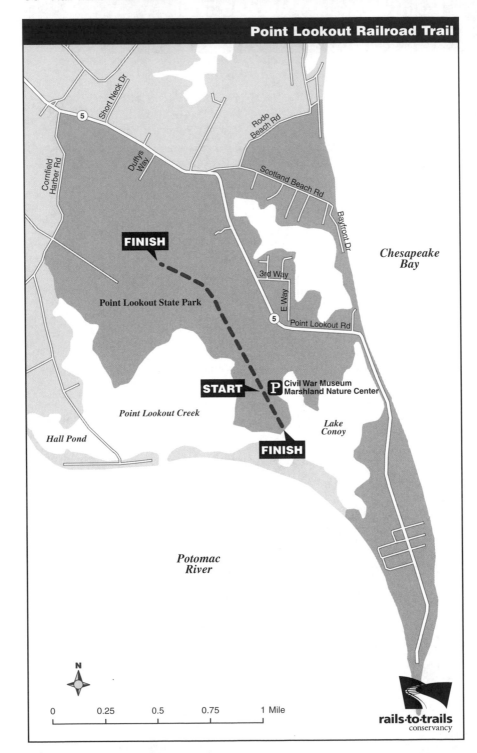

Point Lookout Railroad Trail

Short Neck Dr

5

Rodo Beach Rd

Cornfield Harber Rd

Duffys Way

Scotland Beach Rd

Bayfront Dr

Chesapeake Bay

FINISH

3rd Way

Point Lookout State Park

E Way

5

Point Lookout Rd

START

P Civil War Museum
Marshland Nature Center

Point Lookout Creek

Lake Conoy

Hall Pond

FINISH

Potomac River

N

0   0.25   0.5   0.75   1 Mile

rails·to·trails
conservancy

Turning left at the nature center will take you along a short (less than a quarter mile) stretch of trail where waterfowl and other wildlife viewing is abundant. The trail's end is a rewarding one, with beautiful views of Lake Conoy and the Point Lookout Creek. Late-summer visitors may be treated to migrating monarch butterflies, and if you are on the trail during the spring or fall, be sure to watch for migratory birds.

DIRECTIONS

From Interstate 495, take MD Route 4 south until you cross the Solomons Island Bridge. After the bridge, turn left at the first traffic light onto MD Route 235, heading south. Follow this into a small town called Ridge and turn left at the blinking red light onto MD Route 5, heading south. Follow Route 5 as far as it will go (it takes a sharp right turn as you approach the 5-mile mark) all the way to Point Lookout State Park. In the off-season, stop at the park headquarters to get a code to open the gate to the camping area. After you pass the headquarters office, take your first right into the camping area. After passing the gate, take your first right and then bear left to campsites 26-20, where you will access a parking lot that is adjacent to the trail entrance.

Contact: Point Lookout State Park
11175 Point Lookout Road
Scotland, MD 20687
(301) 872-5688
www.dnr.state.md.us/publiclands/southern/
pointlookout.html

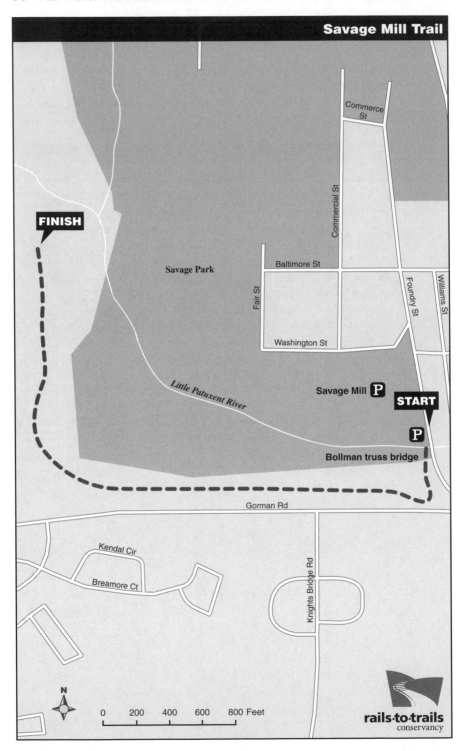

Savage Mill Trail

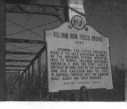

T he Savage Mill Trail in Savage Park travels along the rolling Patuxent River through the grounds of an old cotton mill. In the early 1800s, Savage was a major manufacturing center, harnessing power produced by the falls on the Little and Middle Patuxent rivers. Near the trailhead stands an 1822 textile mill, today renovated as a shopping center where you can buy antiques or grab a picnic lunch to enjoy on the pleasant 1-mile trail.

The trail begins at an old Bollman truss bridge, an iron structure used exclusively by the Baltimore and Ohio Railroad. Built in 1869, the bridge was moved to Savage in 1887. Though the company built about 100 of these bridges before 1873, this is the country's only remaining Bollman bridge of this design. The trail's designers left the train tracks in place on one side of the bridge, so you can imagine the train passing beside you as you ride or walk over this piece of history.

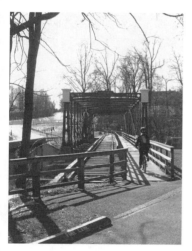

A bicyclist crosses a Bollman truss bridge—a style developed specifically for use on the Baltimore and Ohio Railroad.

Most of the trail is paved and flat, but the surface changes to gravel and then dirt before it ends abruptly in the middle of the woods. Although you are very near a major highway and the bustle of the shopping center, the music of the river rolling over large boulders and the white oaks surrounding the trail create the impression that you're in the wilderness. It's easy to stop and savor the natural oasis at one of the trail's many picnic tables.

The Savage Mill Trail is part of a larger, 20-mile system of pathways through Howard County. For a more challenging trip, hit the Patuxent Branch Trail (page 53), which begins a few blocks away.

Location
Howard County

Endpoints
Foundry Street to
Savage Park

Mileage
1

Roughness Index
1

Surface
Gravel, asphalt, dirt

DIRECTIONS

From Interstate 95, take MD Route 32 (Patuxent Parkway) east to merge onto US Route 1 (Baltimore Washington Blvd.), heading south. Turn right on Gorman Road, and then turn left on Foundry Street. The Savage Mill parking lot is on your left.

Contact: Howard County Recreation and Parks Department
7120 Oakland Mills Road
Columbia, MD 21046
(410) 313-4687
www.co.ho.md.us/RAP/RAP_HomePage.htm

Western Maryland Rail Trail

Plan a full day (or two) for your visit to the Western Maryland Rail Trail, a 22-mile paved route that will take you through several eras of American history.

You can access this trail from many points, but the main trailhead is in the quaint town of Hancock (population 1750). Stop here for food, drinks, antique shopping, to stay the night, or just to wander around the historical downtown, which once served as the frontier of Maryland and frequently was visited by George Washington, among other notables.

From the trailhead in Hancock, you can head east or west along the trail, about 10 miles in either direction. Whichever direction you choose, expect to pass fields and wooded groves. You will also parallel the Chesapeake and Ohio Canal and its 185-mile unpaved towpath, which was used to transport coal from Cumberland, Maryland, to the port of Georgetown in Washington, DC, from 1828 until 1924. The route's historical sites include the canal's locks and lock houses.

The eastern portion is blessed with magnificent views of the Potomac River. Large rock outcroppings

Location
Washington
County

Endpoints
Big Pool
(Fort Frederick
State Park) to
Pearre (Old Pearre
Rail Station)

Mileage
22

**Roughness
Index**
1

Surface
Asphalt

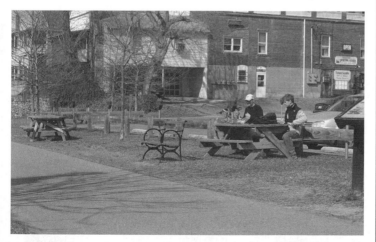

The Western Maryland Rail Trail runs adjacent to the Chesapeake and Ohio Canal for much of its journey, and shares the same historical highlights along the way.

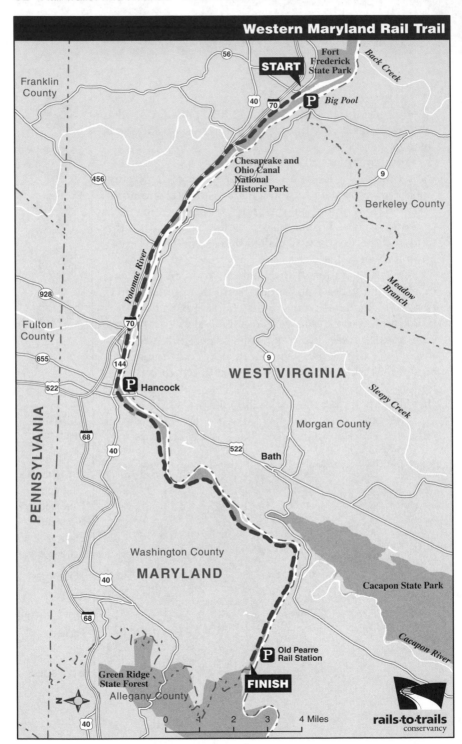

Western Maryland Rail Trail

Franklin County

56

START

Fort Frederick State Park

Back Creek

40 70

P *Big Pool*

Chesapeake and Ohio Canal National Historic Park

9

Berkeley County

456

Potomac River

928

70

Meadow Branch

Fulton County

655

144

522

P Hancock

9

WEST VIRGINIA

Sleepy Creek

PENNSYLVANIA

68

40

522

Bath

Morgan County

Washington County

MARYLAND

Cacapon State Park

40

68

Cacapon River

P Old Pearre Rail Station

Green Ridge State Forest

Allegany County

FINISH

N

40

0   2   3   4 Miles

rails·to·trails
conservancy

will catch your attention, as will the ruins of the Round Top Cement Mill, which was built in the 1830s and was Hancock's largest employer during the Civil War. To the west and just past downtown Hancock, you can buy trailside snacks from the family-owned Hepburn Orchards Fruit Market where, in the 1920s, more than 5000 surrounding acres were planted with fruit trees. Traveling a little farther, you will find historical markers for Little Pool and Park Head cemeteries. Be on the lookout for deer and wild turkey that are not phased by the loud traffic nearby.

To vary your route, and maximize your scenery, take the Western Maryland Rail Trail in one direction and loop back on the Chesapeake & Ohio Canal National Historical Park towpath.

DIRECTIONS

To reach the eastern end of the trail in Fort Frederick State Park, from Interstate 70, take exit 12 to MD Route 56 and head east toward Big Pool. The trail parking lot is across the street from the post office.

To reach Hancock from Interstate 70, take exit 3 and travel west on MD Route 144 for 1.4 miles. There is parking at Hancock Station, just off Main Street.

To begin at the western end of the trail in Pearre, from Interstate 68, take exit 77 and head south on Woodmont Road, which will intersect with the trail at Pearre Road. Parking is available.

Contact: Western Maryland Rail Trail
C/O Fort Frederick State Park
11100 Fort Frederick Road
Big Pool, MD 21711
(301) 842-2155
www.westernmarylandrailtrail.org/WMRT/

Virginia

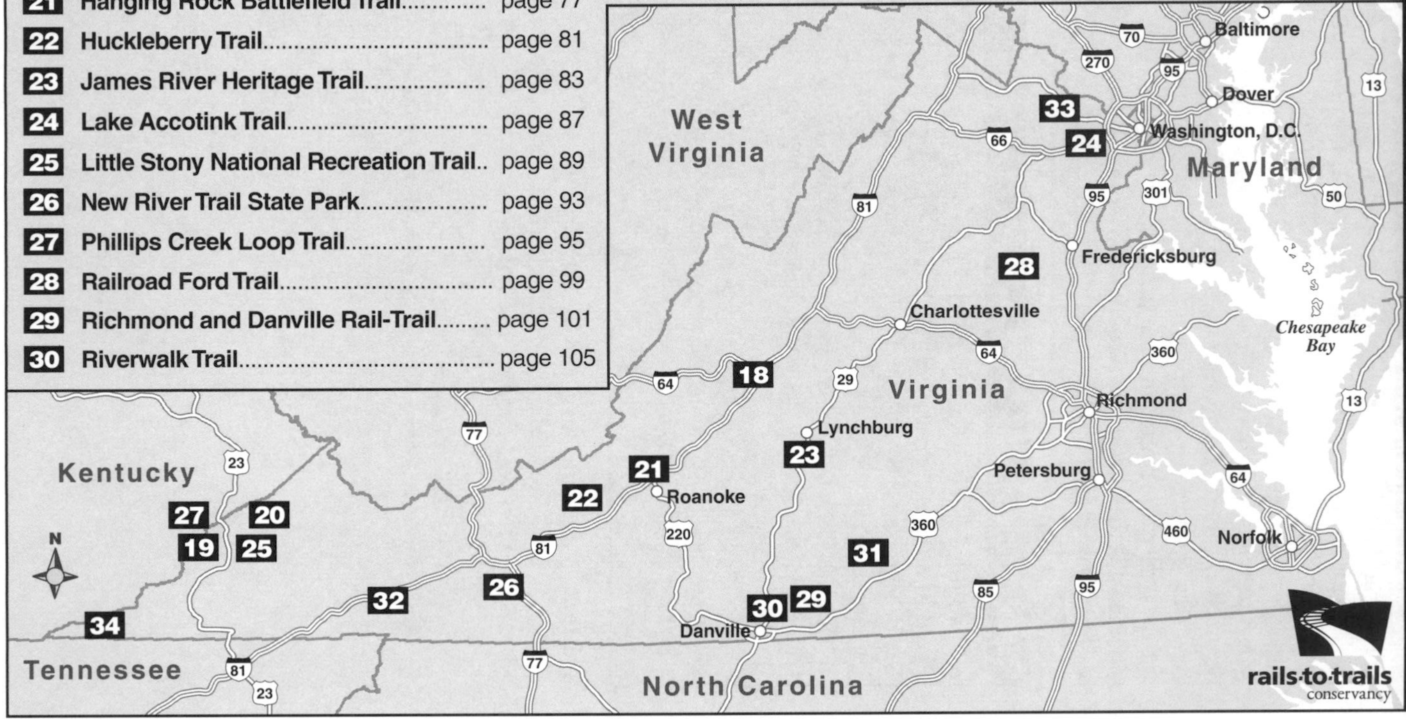

West Virginia
Virginia
Maryland
Kentucky
Tennessee
North Carolina
Baltimore
Dover
Washington, D.C.
Fredericksburg
Charlottesville
Richmond
Lynchburg
Roanoke
Petersburg
Norfolk
Danville
Chesapeake Bay
70
270
95
66
81
301
50
13
64
29
360
77
23
220
460
85
N
rails-to-trails conservancy

Virginia

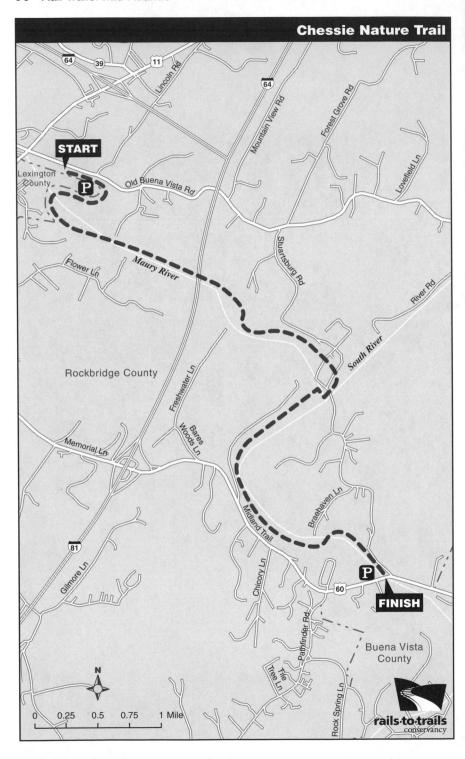

Chessie Nature Trail

Chessie Nature Trail

The pedestrian-only Chessie Nature Trail travels through breathtaking rural Virginia countryside, following mile markers left behind by the Chesapeake & Ohio Railroad that ran this route. Don't be surprised if you find yourself sharing the trail with a wide array of birds and small mammals. There are some large mammals, too. Expect to see a few cattle grazing in the meadows that border the trail. (You may also pass cattle gates, which can be tricky to get around sometimes, but they do not indicate that the trail is closed.)

The trail begins along VA Route 631 in Lexington and follows the northern bank of the Maury River for the first 3.7 miles, while alternating between lush forested areas and farmland. There is a break in the trail at the river, where the former railroad bridge has been removed. To navigate around this, follow Stuartsburg Road (located right next to the trail) south for a half mile before taking a right onto Old Shepard Road and reconnecting to the trail.

The final 2.5 miles meet back up with the river for the remainder of the trail. While the trail passes some

Location
Rockbridge County

Endpoints
Lexington to
Buena Vista

Mileage
7

Roughness Index
1.5

Surface
Ballast

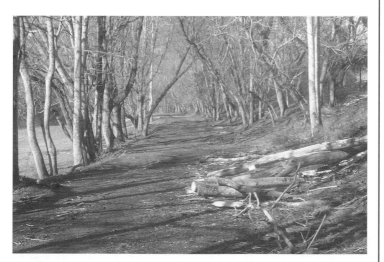

The Chessie Nature Trail runs on the former path of the Richmond & Allegheny Railroad, which later became part of the mammoth Chesapeake & Ohio line.

67

farmland, the final mile hugs a steep cliff along the side of the river on your right. It is quite an impressive finale to this very pleasant walking trail.

DIRECTIONS

To access the Lexington trailhead from the intersection of US Route 11 and Interstate 64 in Lexington, take US 11 south and make a left onto VA Route 631. The trailhead is approximately 1 mile ahead on the right.

To access the Buena Vista trailhead from US Route 60 and Interstate 81 in Lexington, take Route 60 east and make a left on VA Route 608 before Buena Vista. Follow Route 608 for approximately 0.75 mile and look for the trailhead on the left.

Contact: VMI Foundation
PO Box 932
Lexington, VA 24450
(540) 464-7221
www.lexingtonvirginia.com/hiking.htm

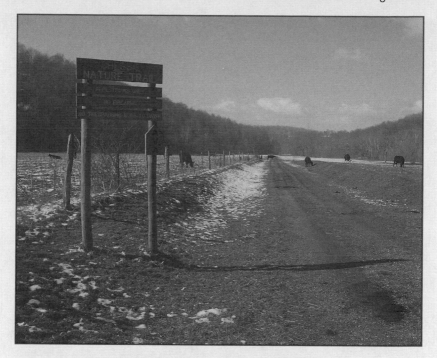

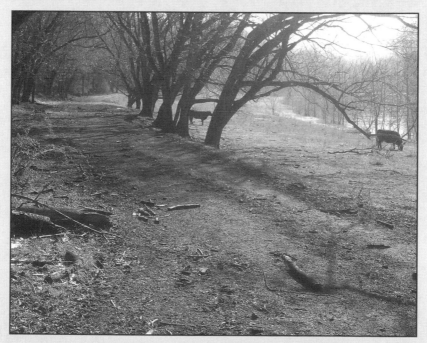

The Chessie Nature Trail cuts through farmland, running adjacent to grazing fields for cows accustomed to sharing their fields with trail users.

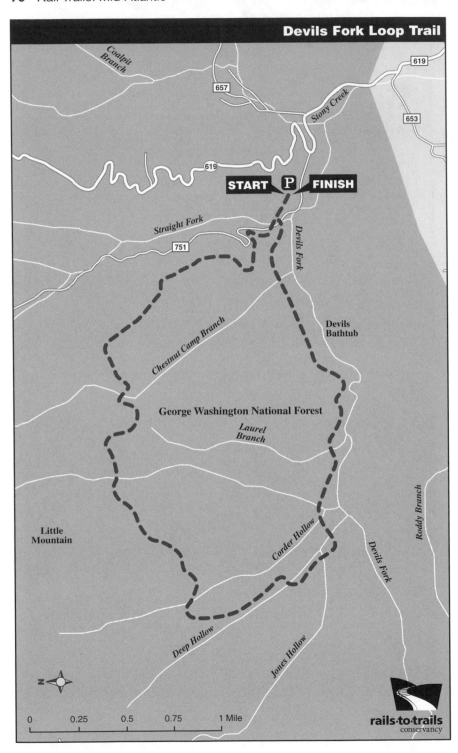

Devils Fork Loop Trail

Devils Fork Loop Trail

Warning

The Devils Fork Loop Trail is extremely challenging, with as many as 18 stream crossings (at the height of the winter thaw), a 1200-foot elevation change, and many opportunities to lose the trail. Be sure to bring enough water for this arduous hike; there are no facilities on or near the trail.

The Devils Fork Loop Trail provides an impressively beautiful—and strenuous—hike through an old-growth hemlock and rhododendron forest. Amazing rock formations, waterfalls, swimming holes, and mountain views give you plenty to see and do, but keep one eye on the trail, as the going can be rough. Although the trail follows yellow blazes for its entire 7 miles, poor maintenance means it is often difficult to find the blazes—and the path, which, in several places, scrambles over large rocks or up very steep cliff faces.

The western leg of the loop follows the Devils Fork, and your first crossing is about one quarter of a mile from the parking lot. Be prepared to get your feet wet. This, like many of the trail's water crossings, has very slippery rocks and seasonally changing water levels. After this, the trail breaks in two directions. The less strenuous

Location
Scott County

Endpoints
George Washington
National Forest

Mileage
7

Roughness Index
3

Surface
Dirt

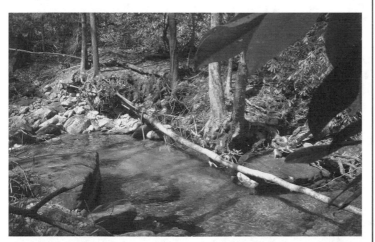

This is one of several stream crossings that make the Devils Fork Loop Trail a challenging but thrilling rail-trail.

route is to the left, following the loop clockwise. This also lets you hit the highlights of the trail much earlier.

The only hint that you are on a rail-trail is the abandoned coal car that sits on the trail about halfway up Little Mountain. In fact, the western side of the loop is the only portion on an old rail bed. This railroad was used to transport logs and coal, and thus the corridor is not as wide as a standard-gauge railway, and the grade is much steeper, which provided the trains with better access to these resources.

The trail's main attraction is Devils Bathtub, located just 1.5 miles from the start. The rushing water of Devils Fork shoots out of the soft sandstone and swirls quickly through this stone luge, plummeting into a beautiful pool of blue-green water. Another trail highlight, shortly after Devils Bathtub, is the 50-foot waterfall at the mouth of Corder Hollow.

The trail enters a very different landscape as you leave the Devils Fork and begin hiking along the ridges of several mountains. The forest has little underbrush and the path can be easily lost.

Your adventure concludes on an old logging road with about a mile of steep switchbacks to the loop's end, where you cross Devils Fork for the last time. There are primitive camping facilities near the parking lot. You can continue hiking by taking the Straight Fork Ridge Trail (1.8 miles) via the parking lot. The scenery on Straight Fork Ridge is similar to the Devils Fork Loop Trail, but the latter is considered the more interesting hike of the two trails.

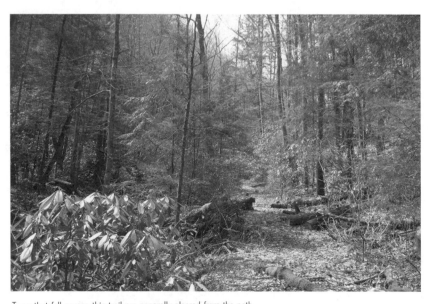

Trees that fall across this trail are generally cleared from the path.

DIRECTIONS

From US Alternate Hwy. 58, take VA Route 72 south toward Fort Blackmore. In Dungannon, Route 72 merges with VA Route 65. Just before they separate in Fort Blackmore, take VA Route 619 to the right.

Alternatively, you can take US Hwy. 23/US Hwy. 58/US Hwy. 421 (Daniel Boone Heritage Hwy.) toward Gate City. In Gate City, continue going straight as the road becomes East Jackson Street and, ultimately, VA Route 71. Head east on Route 71 for a little over a mile. From here, take VA Route 72 to the left toward Fort Blackmore. Shortly after VA Route 65 and VA Route 72 merge, turn left onto VA Route 619.

Once on Route 619, follow VA Route 653 for a short segment, and when they break, look for the DEVILS FORK sign where Route 619 takes a sharp left and becomes Forest Road 619 (there is no street sign). Travel over the one-lane bridge and turn left just before the abandoned white house. Follow this unmarked dirt road to the end, where you will find parking for the trail. The road to the parking lot is very rutted and may not be accessible by all vehicles. You will pass the trailhead on your right just before you reach the parking lot; there are also stairs up to the trail from the parking lot.

Contact: Clinch Ranger District
9416 Darden Drive
Wise, VA 24293
(276) 328-2931
www.fs.fed.us/r8/gwj/clinch

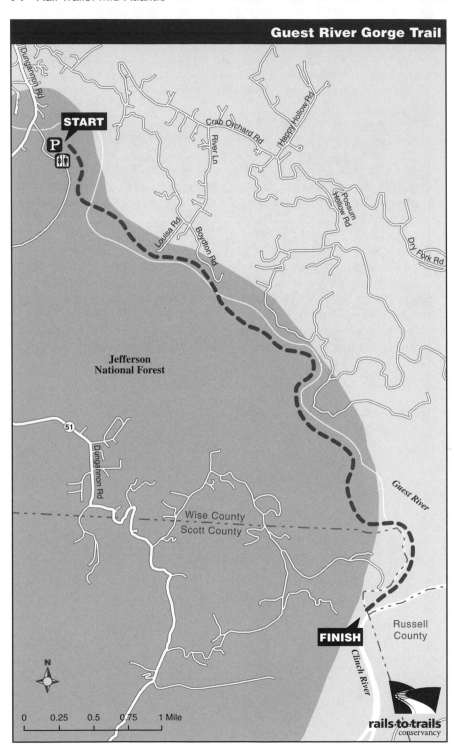

Guest River Gorge Trail

The Guest River Gorge Trail meanders along ancient sandstone cliffs that plunge 400 feet to the pristine waters below. The deep gorge was created as the Guest River, now designated as a state scenic river, tunneled through Stone Mountain on its way toward the Clinch River. The gentle grade of this trail and its gravel surface make it ideal for a comfortable walk or bike ride. Benches along the route offer more than a place to rest: They yield stunning views of crystal-clear currents that, when interrupted sporadically by boulders, turn into impressive rapids.

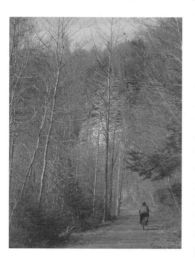

The Guest River Gorge Trail skirts the edge of the vast Jefferson National Forest.

In addition to spectacular Guest River views to the south, the trail offers a trip through the Swede Tunnel, built in 1922. It also crosses three bridges that were built over small creeks to replace the trestles once traveled by rail cars hauling coal mined nearby. Be sure to look for Devil's walking stick, a plant native to the southeast and a member of the ginseng family. This tall and spindly plant produces white blooms during July and August.

Near the end, the trail slopes downhill toward a working rail line across the Guest River. Just before this point, you will see a connection to the Heart of Appalachia Bike Route, which stretches another 125 miles to Burke's Garden in Tazewell County, Virginia. Legend has it that Burke's Garden is so beautiful it was originally sought after as the location for George Washington Vanderbilt's Biltmore Estate, but the people of Burke's Garden refused to sell him any land and thus he built his estate in Ashville, North Carolina, instead.

Location
Scott and Wise counties

Endpoints
Forest Road 2477 in the Jefferson National Forest

Mileage
5.8

Roughness Index
2

Surface
Crushed stone

DIRECTIONS

The Guest River Gorge Trail is an out-and-back trail, so there is only one endpoint. From US Alternative Hwy. 58, head south on VA Route 72 near Coeburn. Travel for 2.3 miles on this curvy, two-lane road. You will pass the Flatwoods Picnic Area on your right, and very soon afterward, you will reach a sign for the Guest River Gorge on your left. Turn left onto this paved road, which is Forest Road 2477, and drive for 1.4 miles until you reach the parking lot. The trailhead is marked with a kiosk at the edge of the parking area.

Contact: Clinch Ranger District
9416 Darden Drive
Wise, VA 24293
(276) 328-2931
www.fs.fed.us/r8/gwj/clinch/

Opened in 1999, the Hanging Rock Battlefield Trail in Salem (just outside of Roanoke) is associated with Southern Virginia's impressive Civil War history. The northern trailhead at Hanging Rock was the site of the 1864 "Hunter's Raid" battle in which General John McCausland's Confederate forces won a substantial victory against the retreating Union army under the command of General David Hunter. The site is marked by a monument along VA Route 311.

The Hanging Rock trailhead is a good place to start your trip. Parking is plentiful, and you can hit the convenience store and gas station next door to stock up on provisions. On the trail, you can absorb the Roanoke Valley's beautiful wooded scenery, as the corridor winds along Mason Creek and Kessler Mill Road.

After passing under Interstate 81, you will soon enter the township of Salem. The trails curves through a residential area, and houses flank the trail until you reach the southern trailhead at Timberview Road. If time permits on your return to the northern trailhead, take a quick jaunt on the short hiking trail at the Hanging Rock trailhead. It meanders along Peter's Creek right up to Interstate 81.

Location
Roanoke County

Endpoints
VA Route 311 to
Kessler Mill Road

Mileage
1.7

**Roughness
Index**
2

Surface
Crushed stone

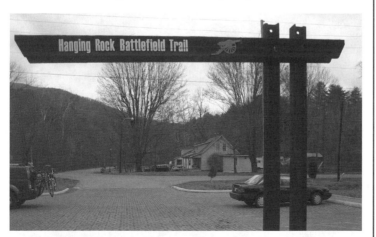

While many rail-trails have a Civil War connection, the Hanging Rock Battlefield Trail is on the actual site of a battle, "Hunter's Raid."

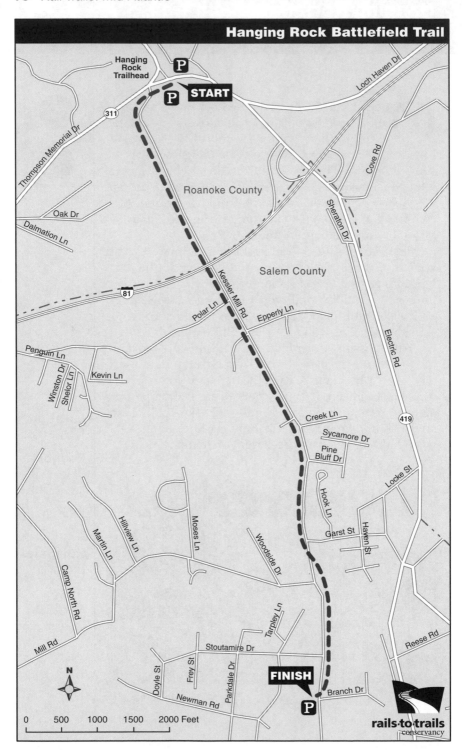

DIRECTIONS

To reach the Hanging Rock trailhead from Interstate 81, take exit 141 to Salem. Turn left onto VA Route 311. The parking area for the Hanging Rock Battlefield Trail is on the left, adjacent to the parking area for the convenience store or across Route 311 at the monument.

To reach the southern terminus from VA Route 419, go west on East Main Street in Salem. At the first light, turn right onto Kessler Mill Road and drive a half mile to the parking lot on the left.

Contact: Roanoke Valley Greenways
PO Box 29800
Roanoke, VA 24018
(540) 387-6060
www.greenways.org

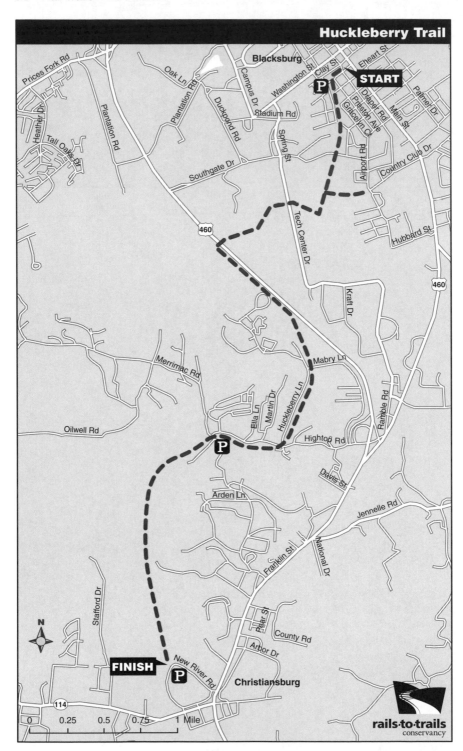

Huckleberry Trail

I n the early 1900s, a train line nicknamed "the Huckleberry" was built to transport coal and provide mail and passenger service to Blacksburg. The line was also used by the Corps cadets at Virginia Polytechnic Institute (more commonly known as Virginia Tech), who unofficially renamed Blacksburg "Huckleberry Junction" due to the abundance of huckleberries that grew along the train line. The huckleberries grew after trees were cleared for railroad construction, and thereafter, the region became famous for delicious pies and jams. Although many of the huckleberries along the trail today have diminished due to increased shade, trail users can find huckleberry bushes planted around trail information kiosks.

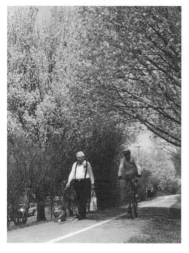

Near the start of the Huckleberry Trail, flowering trees form a canopy for trail users.

The northern trailhead for the Huckleberry Trail is nestled in a residential neighborhood at the Montgomery/Floyd Regional Library in downtown Blacksburg, across from the Virginia Tech campus. You may hear a marching band in the distance or notice a game at the nearby Worsham Field on campus.

As you continue along this meandering trail, you leave the city and enter into rural farmland, passing behind quiet homes and through open fields and pockets of forests. The Coal Miner's Heritage Park at mile 4 displays old mining equipment, just before you reach a railroad bridge over the still-active Norfolk Southern rail line. Unlike most rail-trails, this trail has many gentle curves and slopes—providing diversity in your trail experience. In fact, it is on these steeper sections that the old trains were said to have

Location
Montgomery County

Endpoints
Blacksburg to Christiansburg

Mileage
6.2

Roughness Index
1

Surface
Asphalt

slowed down enough for the cadets to hop from the cars and gather huckleberries before the train gathered more speed. Continue in a southern direction on the trail to reach the trailhead at New River Valley Mall in Christiansburg.

DIRECTIONS

To reach the northern trailhead, take US Hwy. 460 toward Blacksburg and turn onto Main Street (take the US Hwy. 460 Business route), heading north. Turn left on Miller Street, heading southwest, and drive three blocks to Harrell Street, where street parking is available. The trailhead is located in the library parking lot on Miller Street. However, avoid using this lot; towing may be enforced for trail users parked here.

To reach the southern trailhead, take US Hwy. 460 toward Christiansburg, and turn right on VA Route 144 (Peppers Ferry Road). The New River Valley Mall is on the right on New River Road. Follow New River Road, which loops around the mall; trailhead parking is at the back of the mall.

Contact: Montgomery County Government Center
755 Roanoke Street, Suite 2A
Christiansburg, VA 24073
(540) 394-2148
www.montva.com

James River Heritage Trail

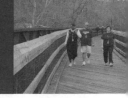

The James River Heritage Trail is one of the premier urban trails in the state, passing through lush forestland as well as the heart of historic, industrial downtown Lynchburg. It also offers multiple easy connections to other trails along the way, and it is well-marked with trail and mileage signs.

The trail begins at the impressively maintained Blackwater Creek Bikeway trailhead, which has a pleasant garden and immaculate facilities. From here, the trail follows an old railroad grade through the Blackwater Creek Natural Area; the first 3-mile section of the trail is called Blackwater Creek Bikeway.

As you descend into the forested canyon that has been carved out by the creek, you will reach a trail junction for the 1.3-mile Kemper Street Station Trail to the south and the 1.7-mile Point of Honor Trail to the north. Both of these paved trails are considered part of the James River Heritage Trail system and are great side trips off the main track.

For the next mile, the trail swings toward downtown and becomes the Lynchburg Riverwalk before crossing

Location
Lynchburg City and
Amherst County

Endpoints
Old Langthorne
Road to Fertilizer
Road

Mileage
9.2

Roughness Index
1

Surface
Asphalt

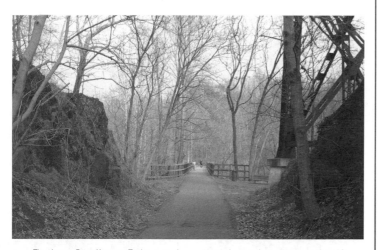

The James River Heritage Trail is part of a greater trail network running more than 12 miles and spanning two counties.

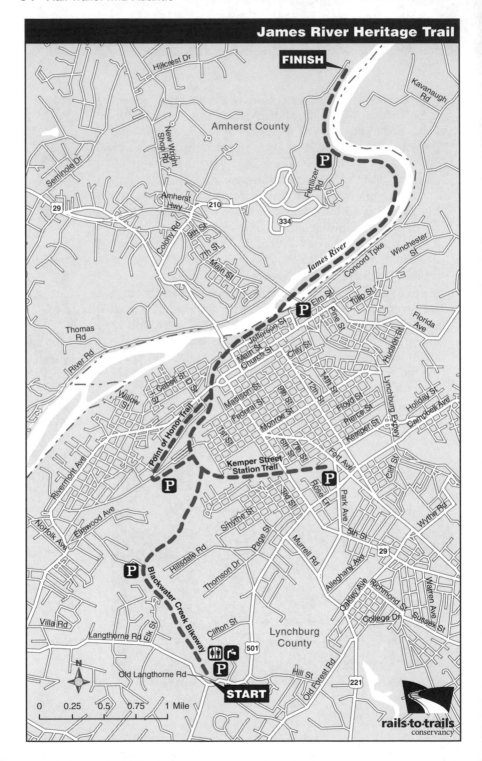

James River Heritage Trail

FINISH

Amherst County

Hillcrest Dr

Kavanaugh Rd

New Wright Shop Rd

Seminole Dr

Colony Rd

Amherst Hwy

29

210

334

9th St

7th St

Main St

James River

Concord Tpke

Winchester St

Elm St

Tulip St

Pine St

Florida Ave

Thomas Rd

River Rd

Willow St

Cabell St

D St

E St

Jefferson St

Main St

Church St

Clay St

Madison St

Federal St

Monroe St

1st St

9th St

12th St

14th St

Floyd St

Pierce St

Kemper St

Lynchburg Expwy

Holiday St

Campbell Ave

Point of Honor Trail

Kemper Street Station Trail

6th St

7th St

5th St

Fort Ave

Rose Ln

Park Ave

5th St

Cliff St

Wythe Rd

Riverfront Ave

Norfolk Ave

Elmwood Ave

Hillsdale Rd

Smyrne St

Page St

Murrell Rd

29

Alleghany Ave

Blackwater Creek Bikeway

Thomson Dr

Clifton St

Lynchburg County

501

Oakley Ave

Richmond St

College Dr

Sussex St

Warren Ave

Villa Rd

Langthorne Rd

Elk St

Old Langthorne Rd

Hill St

Old Forest Rd

221

N

START

0   0.25   0.5   0.75   1 Mile

rails-to-trails
conservancy

a spectacular refurbished railroad bridge onto Percival's Island. The trail traverses the mile-long island before crossing a second former rail bridge to the eastern shore of the James River. It continues for another 2 miles along the river's edge until its end less than a mile past the last trail access point located off of Fertilizer Road. When you reach the endpoint, the railroad corridor clearly continues, and there are plans to extend this wonderful trail.

DIRECTIONS

To reach the Blackwater Creek Bikeway trailhead from the Lynchburg Expressway, go north on US Hwy. 501, which becomes Langthorne Road. Be on the lookout for a quick right turn onto Old Langthorne Road; the trailhead is on the left.

To reach the Fertilizer Road trailhead from the Lynchburg Expressway, take VA Route 210 east to Fertilizer Road and turn right to follow it all the way the trailhead for parking.

Contact: Lynchburg City Parks
301 Grove Street
Lynchburg, VA 24501
(434) 455-5858
www.lynchburgva.gov/home/index.asp?page=86

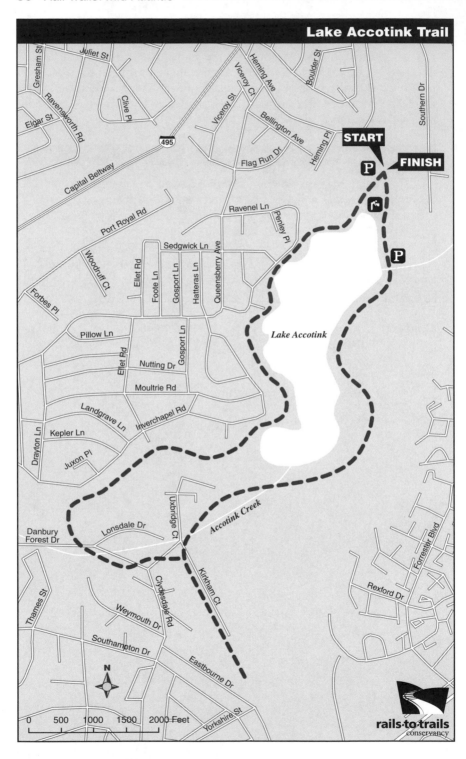

Lake Accotink Trail

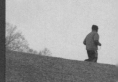

In the suburban community of Springfield in Northern Virginia, Lake Accotink Park provides a wilderness escape amid the city surroundings. The nearly 500-acre park features picnic areas, miniature golf, an antique carousel, a 55-acre lake with canoe and kayak rentals, and of course, trails.

The Lake Accotink Trail follows part of the former rail bed of the Orange and Alexandria Railroad, along which soldiers and materials were transported during the Civil War. Historical markers outline the railroad's history and help mark the entry to the park. At the trail's start, it's impossible to miss the still-operating trestle bridge running high above Accotink Creek. The creek's dam, constructed more then 50 years ago, created a popular fishing hole. As you leave the picnic and boat-rental area behind, the trail shoots up a short, steep hill toward the woods surrounding the lake.

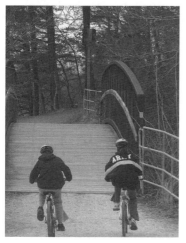

Lake Accotink Trail is a popular destination for Northern Virginians seeking a little woodland respite.

The first half of this route hugs the lake's curves as it travels deeper into the small woodlands preserve that provides shade and wonderful views of marshland and the lake. When you reach the fork in the road at the trail's midpoint, either continue straight to get another 0.75-mile jaunt on the rail-trail before it dead-ends at Rolling Road, or follow the trail marker indicating a right turn to loop back to your starting point. This 4.5-mile option takes you down a short hill and onto neighborhood sidewalks for three or four blocks as you pass an elementary school before you return to the park.

Location
Fairfax County

Endpoints
Marina at Lake Accotink Park

Mileage
4.5

Roughness Index
2

Surface
Crushed stone, gravel, asphalt

On the main route, several stairs lead downhill to a bridge and back to the Lake Accotink Trail, which circles around the other side of the lake, to the creek and surrounding marshland. Your round trip will end with a wonderful view of the antique carousel and geese swimming in the shallow lake waters.

DIRECTIONS

From Washington, DC, take Interstate 395 south. This turns into Interstate 95 south at Springfield. Take the Old Keene Mill Road exit (VA Route 644) west toward Springfield. Turn slightly right onto Backlick Road and then turn left onto Highland Street. Follow Highland Street through a neighborhood and then turn slightly right onto Accotink Park Road. Follow this road through the park and past the trestle bridge to arrive at the parking lot.

Contact: Fairfax County Park Authority
7500 Accotink Park Road
Springfield, VA 22150
(703) 569-3464
www.fairfaxcounty.gov/parks/accotink

Little Stony National Recreation Trail

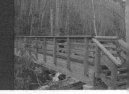

If you're looking for an easy trip, the Little Stony National Recreation Trail in Jefferson National Forest is the perfect alternative to the nearby Devils Fork Loop (see page 71). Devils Fork Loop is gorgeous, but it includes a strenuous and often wet climb. Little Stony, on the other hand, offers similarly beautiful views within a mere 2.8 miles, and its footbridges save you from cold, slippery water crossings. You can also take breaks from the trail's 600-foot ascent by resting at the bridges high above the rushing currents and below the hemlock canopy.

Starting at Hanging Rock Picnic Area, follow the yellow blazes marking the trail, which snakes along Little Stony Creek. The trail is rather narrow in areas where it climbs in elevation and travels over boulders, and the slope is steep for a rail-trail, but the exhilarating views are worth every step. Within a half-mile of the northern trailhead, you will find a sanctuary-like viewing platform across from a 40-foot waterfall. Thick, waxy leaves of rhododendron and mountain laurel frame the white veil of water, and if you visit in May or June, you'll likely catch the spectacular blooms of these plants.

Location
Scott County

Endpoints
Hanging Rock Picnic Area to Little Stony Falls in the Jefferson National Forest

Mileage
2.8

Roughness Index
3

Surface
Dirt

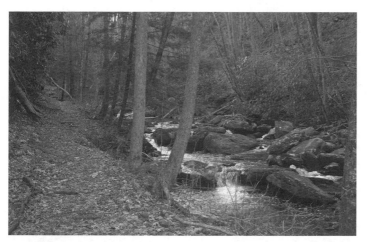

Tucked in the Jefferson National Forest, this trail crisscrosses the Little Stony Creek and passes a 40-foot waterfall.

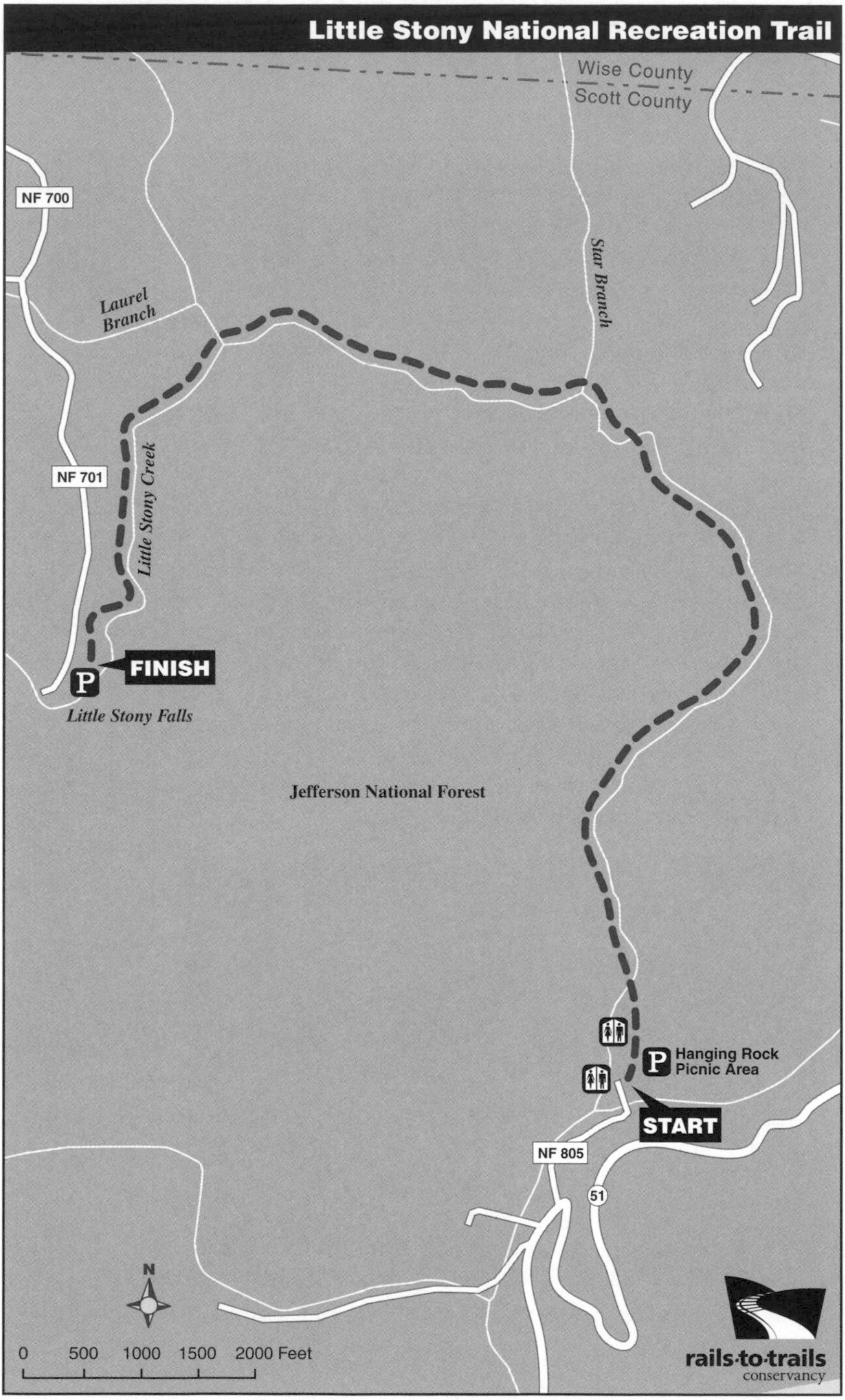

Little Stony National Recreation Trail

Wise County

Scott County

NF 700

Star Branch

Laurel
Branch

NF 701

Little Stony Creek

P **FINISH**

Little Stony Falls

Jefferson National Forest

P Hanging Rock
Picnic Area

START

NF 805

51

N

0   500   1000   1500   2000 Feet

rails·to·trails
conservancy

Continue uphill to find two more impressive waterfalls. Several hundred feet beyond these, you will arrive at the Little Stony Falls parking area, where the 16-mile Chief Benge Scout Trail picks up from Forest Road 701.

DIRECTIONS

To access the Hanging Rock Picnic Area from US Alternative Route 58, head south on VA Route 72 near Coeburn. Travel for approximately 7 miles to the Hanging Rock Picnic Area. A sign marks the trailhead.

The upper trailhead, north of Hanging Rock, is a bit more complicated to find. Fortunately, the forest roads that you need to take are peppered with signs to Little Stony Falls. From the junction of VA Route 72 south and US Alternative Route 58, travel south on VA 72 to the minor VA Route 664. Go west on VA 664 for about 1 mile to Forest Road 700. From there, follow signs to Little Stony Falls.

Contact: Clinch Ranger District
9416 Darden Drive
Wise, VA 24293
(276) 328-2931
www.fs.fed.us/r8/gwj/clinch

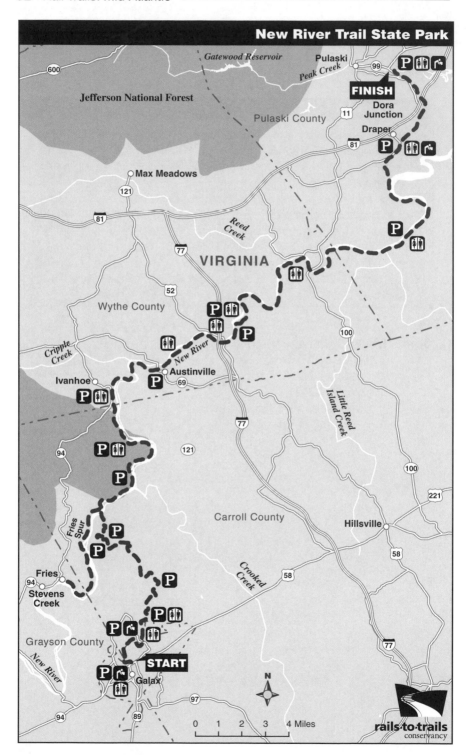

New River Trail State Park

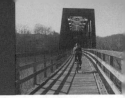

S outhern Virginia's New River Trail is one of America's premier rail-trails and has been designated as an official National Recreation Trail by the US Department of the Interior. It is also a state park. The highlight and namesake of this magnificent trail is the 36-mile section running through Grayson, Carroll, Wythe, and Pulaski counties along the New River, the oldest river in the US. In 1986, the Norfolk and Southern Railroad donated this old railroad corridor, which originally served to supply the once expanding iron industry to the Commonwealth of Virginia.

The best place to start a trip along this trail is at its southern terminus in Galax. Note that from this direction, the mileage markers count down beginning at the 57-mile marker. A large part of the trail is uphill if you start at the northern terminus at Dora Junction along Interstate 81.

The Galax trailhead, which features an old red caboose, has plenty of parking. From here, you follow Chestnut Creek along the 12-mile Galax to Fries Junction section. At mile marker 38, you'll encounter the beautiful

Location
Pulaski, Carroll, Grayson, and Wythe counties

Endpoints
Galax to Pulaski

Mileage
57

Roughness Index
1.5

Surface
Crushed stone

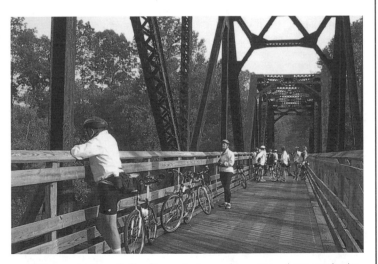

Riders peer down over the New River, an ironic name for a waterway that is considered to be the oldest river in the US.

Fries Junction trestle bridge crossing the New River. Just across the bridge, you have the option of taking a pleasant excursion to Fries, a 12-mile round trip. This 6-mile spur is included in the trail's 57-mile total length.

The remaining 39 miles proceeds north along the peacefully flowing New River as it runs through Cripple Creek Junction, Foster Falls, and Allisonia. The trail is isolated for much of this journey, so if you are on this stretch, be sure to carry all necessary supplies in case of an emergency or quick bike repair. Along the way, you'll see many railroading highlights, including cavernous tunnels, steep dams, and trestle bridges—including the impressive 950-foot Hiawassee trestle around mile marker 8. The trail finally concludes at Dora Junction, near the town of Pulaski, where you will be able to find all your post-trail amenities.

DIRECTIONS

To the Galax trailhead, take Interstate 77 to the US Hwy. 221/US Hwy. 58 exit (exit 14) toward Hillsville/Galax. The trailhead is located on the right, where Route 58 crosses Chestnut Creek.

To reach the Dora Junction trailhead in Pulaski from Interstate 81, take VA Route 99 west for 2 miles toward Xaloy. Turn right on Xaloy Way and look for the trailhead on the right.

You can also access the trail in Fries: Take Interstate 77 to the US Hwy. 221/US Hwy. 58 exit (exit 14) toward Hillsville/Galax. Turn right at Cliffview Road/VA Route 721 to Fries. Route 721 becomes Fries Road before crossing the New River. As you come into town, turn left on Dalton Road. The trailhead is at the bottom of the hill; the trail signs are impossible to miss. Parking is available near the town park on Riverview Ave.

Contact: New River Trail State Park
176 Orphanage Drive
Foster Falls, VA 24360
(276) 699-6778
www.dcr.state.va.us/parks/newriver.htm

Phillips Creek Loop Trail

The short, relatively easy Phillips Creek Loop (also known as the Pine Mountain Trail) begins in a pleasant recreation area that is open May 15 to September 15 and provides paid parking, swimming, restrooms, and secluded picnic areas. The trail is open for hiking all year, but since the area is gated (and the restrooms are closed) in the off-season, you must park your car at the gate and walk about a half mile to the trailhead.

From the information kiosk, follow a footbridge into a forest that includes thickets of rhododendron and a stand of white pines. On the first half of the loop, you will walk alongside Phillips Creek. Keep your eyes open for an old hunting camp used by Native Americans, as well as the site of an old moonshine still located across the creek. These sites are not well-marked. Since they are not obvious, consider calling the Clinch Ranger District (276-328-2931) to order an informational brochure explaining the various points of interest along the trail.

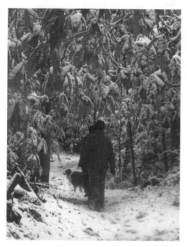

In winter, the Phillips Creek Loop Trail is a wonderland in a forest of rhododendrons.

At the far end of the loop is a scenic waterfall along a sandstone cliff. The trek back to the parking lot travels on an old railroad bed that was used in the late 1800s and early 1900s to haul logs.

Location
Wise County

Endpoints
Phillips Creek
Recreation Area

Mileage
1

Roughness Index
3

Surface
Dirt

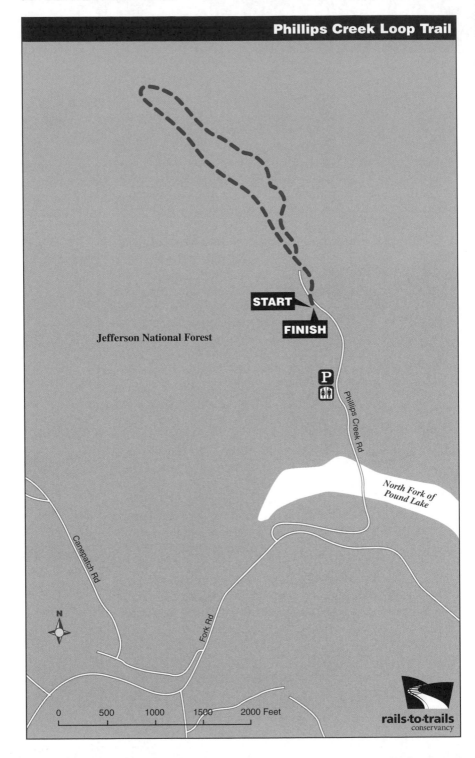

Phillips Creek Loop Trail

START

FINISH

Jefferson National Forest

P

Phillips Creek Rd

North Fork of Pound Lake

Canepatch Rd

Fork Rd

N

0   500   1000   1500   2000 Feet

rails·to·trails
conservancy

DIRECTIONS

To access this trail, take US Hwy. 23 north near Norton toward Pound. As you approach Pound, stay on Hwy. 23 (do not turn onto Business 23). Turn west onto VA Route 671 and follow it for about 5.5 miles to the marked Phillips Creek Recreation Area. The trailhead is located all the way down the gravel road, past the swimming area and all the picnic areas. It is marked by a footbridge and information kiosk that reads PINE MOUNTAIN TRAIL.

Contact: Clinch Ranger District
9416 Darden Drive
Wise, VA 24293
(276) 328-2931
www.fs.fed.us/r8/gwj/clinch

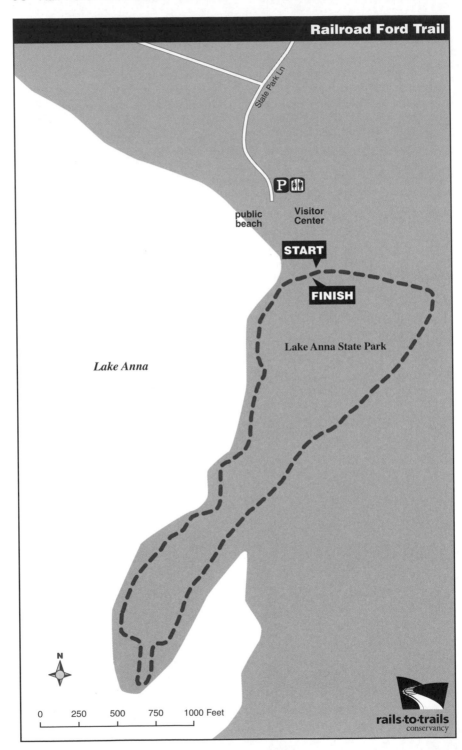

Railroad Ford Trail

State Park Ln

public beach

Visitor Center

START

FINISH

Lake Anna State Park

Lake Anna

N

0 250 500 750 1000 Feet

rails·to·trails
conservancy

Railroad Ford Trail

The Railroad Ford Trail is located in beautiful Lake Anna State Park in Spotsylvania County between Washington, DC, and Richmond, Virginia. The park boasts 2463 acres with 11 trails, swimming, boating, fishing, horseback riding, and camping. The park is open daily from 8 AM to dusk.

This loop trail (which is rough but wheelchair-accessible) is a section of the original 17.5-mile rail corridor that was established in 1917 to support the war effort in Europe. The railroad was used to transport ore from Holladay Mine, 5 miles north, to Allah Cooper Mine, 7 miles down the track. Lead and zinc were extracted from the ore and transported 10 miles to Mineral, Virginia, where they were then shipped on the C&O Railroad to northern factories to make bullets and shell cartridges.

Today, visitors will find a beautiful walking trail, sun-dappled by a tree canopy. To find the trailhead, follow the sidewalk past the visitor center and boat-rental area. The trail begins at the marker where the sidewalk ends. From the trail marker, bear right to begin your walk along this loop. The 0.75 miles takes you along a packed dirt path that runs parallel to the lake.

Location
Spotsylvania County

Endpoints
Lake Anna State Park Visitor Center

Mileage
1.6

Roughness Index
2

Surface
Dirt

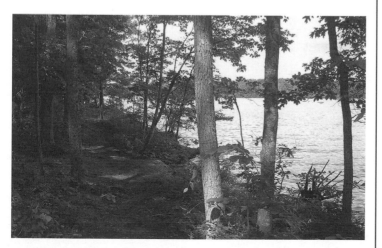

Looking out over Lake Anna's swimming and boating area on the Railroad Ford Trail

Take in the rich lake views and try out the many short paths to reach the water's edge, where you can access one of the many benches along this stretch. When the trail bears left after less than a mile, it becomes wider, elevated, and flat. It's easy to imagine the route of the original railroad corridor here, and, indeed, a historical railroad sign is also posted along this section. As you conclude your walk, the trail intersects with the Glenora Trail, a wide equestrian trail. Turn left at this intersection for a short stretch that completes the loop.

DIRECTIONS

From Washington, DC, or Richmond, Virginia, take Interstate 95 to the Thornburg exit (exit 118). Go west on VA Route 208 and follow signs to Lake Anna State Park. Drive approximately 11 miles on Route 208. After passing a high school on your left, the road takes a sharp left turn. You will see a pretty white farm house on the corner and a sign for the state park indicating you should follow Route 208 and bear left. Go approximately 7 more miles and turn right onto VA Route 601. Travel 3.3 miles and turn left into Lake Anna State Park. Shortly after the park entrance, you will have to pay a park entrance fee of $3 on weekdays and $4 on weekends. Continue following the main entrance road until it ends at the beach and main parking area. At the back of the parking lot, you will see the Lake Anna State Park Visitor Center (open Memorial Day to Labor Day). Follow the sidewalk past the visitor center and boat-rental area to the trailhead.

Contact: Lake Anna State Park
6800 Lawyers Road
Spotsylvania, VA 22553
(540) 854-5503
www.dcr.virginia.gov

Richmond and Danville Rail-Trail

The Richmond and Danville Railroad was an important transportation corridor for the Confederacy during the Civil War, linking the Confederate capital of Richmond with Southside, the area between the James River and the North Carolina border, where hospitals, prisons, and supply depots were located. Jefferson Davis and the Confederate army took the route of this railroad line when they retreated from Richmond near the end of the war. They also used it to carry war materials and Union prisoners.

Today, 5.5 miles of this historical corridor, which eventually became part of the Norfolk Southern Railway system, is the scenic Richmond and Danville Rail-Trail. Also called the Ringgold Trail, this trail was opened in January 2001. It travels past farmlands and through light woods, providing a flat route for a walk or bike ride in the rural Virginia countryside on the outskirts of Danville.

Start your trip at the western trailhead, and in only 1 mile you will reach a wetland area with prime waterfowl watching. The ride is comfortable for bicyclists or walkers of all ages, and is wheelchair accessible. You can

Location
Pittsylvania County

Endpoints
Ringgold Depot
Road to Kerns
Church Road

Mileage
5.5

Roughness Index
2

Surface
Crushed stone

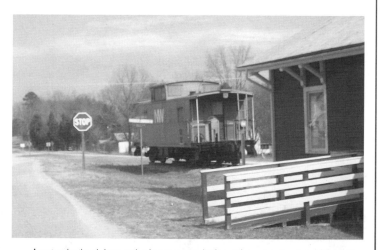

A restored railroad depot and caboose are on display at the eastern terminus of the trail.

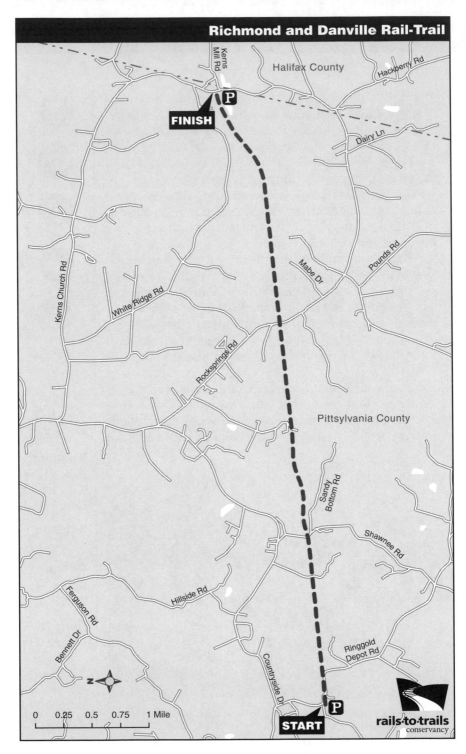

brush up on your Civil War history as well; plaques along the way detail significant events that happened near the rail-trail. For those looking for evidence of the trail's railroading past, the eastern trailhead houses a restored railroad depot and an old red caboose.

DIRECTIONS

From Danville, take US Hwy. 58 east for approximately 2.5 miles, and then head north on State Route 62 (Ringgold Depot Road) for 3 miles. The western trailhead is located on the south side of Ringgold Depot Road.

To access the eastern trailhead, continue east on Hwy. 58 for an additional 3.75 miles, and then head north on Hackberry Road for 3.25 miles. The trailhead is located west of Hackberry Road (Kerns Church Road), near the intersection of Kerns Mill Road.

Contact: Dan River Trail Association
PO Box 1375
(804) 822-5725
www.danrta.homestead.com

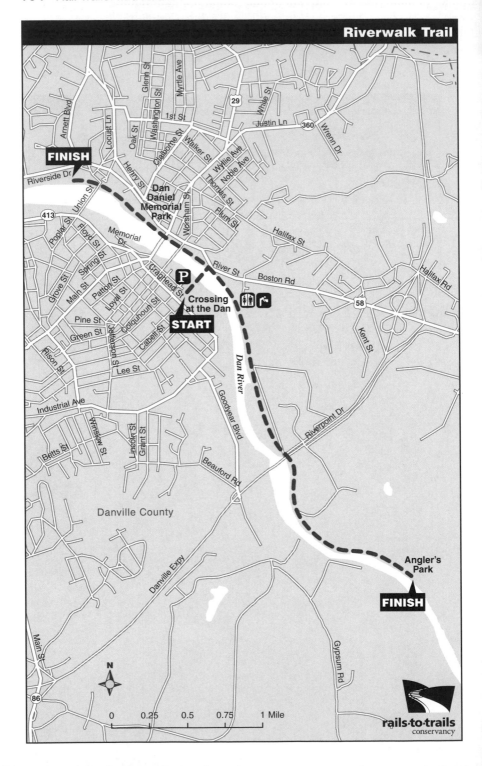

Riverwalk Trail

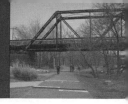

The 6.5-mile, paved Riverwalk Trail is part of Danville's expanding network of trails. This scenic pathway along the Dan River connects industry, beautiful parks, and natural areas. It travels through some of the most important and historical Civil War regions of southern Virginia.

Throughout the Civil War, Danville functioned as a staging area for many battles. Some of its old tobacco warehouses were turned into Civil War prisons and the city was the last capital of the Confederate States of America, after Richmond was captured by the Union army.

The trail's recommended starting point is at the Crossing at the Dan trailhead in historical downtown Danville, alongside a renovated tobacco warehouse and the active Amtrak station located in the Science Center. From here, you'll cross the Dan River on a restored 1856 railroad bridge. At the other side, you can go east or west. If you turn left (west), the trail follows the river upstream for about 1 mile along the river until it reaches the beautiful overlook at Union Street Bridge.

Location
Danville County

Endpoints
Crossing at the Dan to Angler's Park to Union Street Bridge

Mileage
6.5

Roughness Index
1

Surface
Asphalt

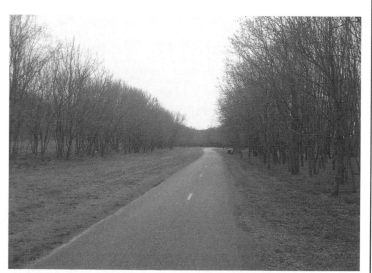

The Riverwalk Trail traces an easy path along the Dan River.

However, the best part of the trail lies to the right, on the eastern side. From here, the riverside trail will take you on an enjoyable trip through the many beautiful parks and natural areas adjacent to the Dan River. You'll see a variety of wildlife, including a goose or two using the trail themselves. Once you pass Dan Daniel Memorial Park, the trail continues to wind along the river until it concludes at Angler's Park. At the Angler's Park trailhead, you have the option of continuing on the trail segment toward Danville Regional Airport.

DIRECTIONS

To reach the Crossing at the Dan, from South VA Business Route 58 in downtown Danville, take Main Street south across the Dan River and make a left on Craghead Street. Follow that for approximately five blocks until you see signs for the train station on the left. The trailhead will be on the far side of the parking lot.

Contact: Danville Parks, Recreation, and Tourism
125 Floyd Street
Danville, VA 24541
(434) 799-5200
www.danville-va.gov

Staunton River Battlefield Rail-Trail

This trail, part of Staunton River Battlefield State Park in rural south-central Virginia, follows the corridor of the historic Richmond and Danville Railroad. The primary feature of the trail—a trestle spanning the Staunton River—has a significant place in Civil War history. In 1864, the Union army planned to move into the region and destroy the trestle. If the Union had succeeded, it would have cut off a crucial Confederate supply line leading all the way to Richmond. The story goes that a band of local men held off the Union advancement, preserving the trestle. In addition to the trail and its storied trestle, the park is home to two visitors centers, a museum, a Civil War fort, and a peaceful nature trail.

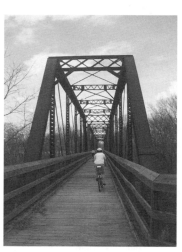

A railroad trestle on the Staunton River Battlefield Rail-Trail

The rail-trail begins by the Clover Visitors Center, near the park entrance. It immediately takes you over the stunning Staunton River Bridge and then through a beautiful open meadow. Two more trestle crossings await—both spanning marshy fields—before the trail's end at the Roanoke Station Visitors Center in Randolph. Although both visitor centers have restroom facilities, water, and parking, the operating hours fluctuate. Be sure to call the state park before heading out.

Location
Charlotte County

Endpoints
Staunton River Battlefield State Park to Randolph

Mileage
1.25

Roughness Index
1

Surface
Ballast

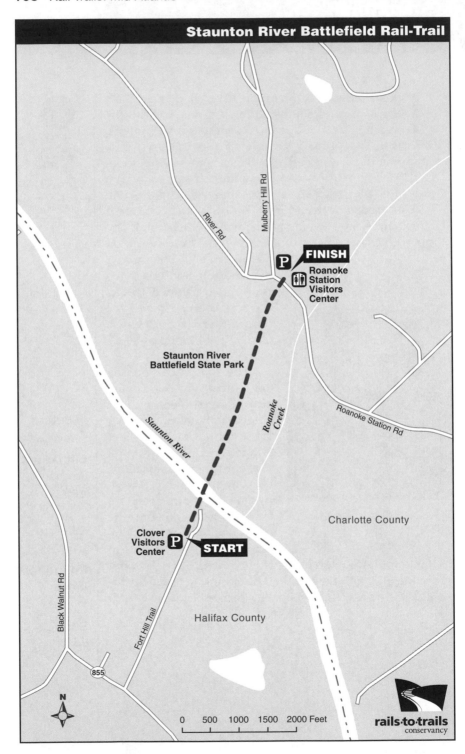

Staunton River Battlefield Rail-Trail

P

FINISH

Roanoke Station Visitors Center

Mulberry Hill Rd

River Rd

Staunton River Battlefield State Park

Roanoke Creek

Staunton River

Roanoke Station Rd

Charlotte County

Clover Visitors Center

P

START

Black Walnut Rd

Fort Hill Trail

855

Halifax County

N

0   500   1000   1500   2000 Feet

rails·to·trails
conservancy

DIRECTIONS

To reach the Clover Visitors Center trailhead from South Boston, take US Hwy. 360 and turn left on VA Route 92 to Clover. Go approximately 5 miles and turn left on VA Route 600. Drive about another 3 miles, look for the sign to the park, and turn right on VA Route 855 into the entrance.

To reach the Roanoke Visitors Center in Randolph from South Boston, take US Hwy. 360 to Branch Road (VA Route 608) and make a left. Follow this to its junction with Roanoke Station Road (VA Route 607) and turn left. Continue all the way to the trailhead on your left in Randolph.

Contact: Staunton River Battlefield State Park
1035 Fort Hill Trail
Randolph, VA 23962
(434) 454-4312
www.stauntonriverbattlefield.org

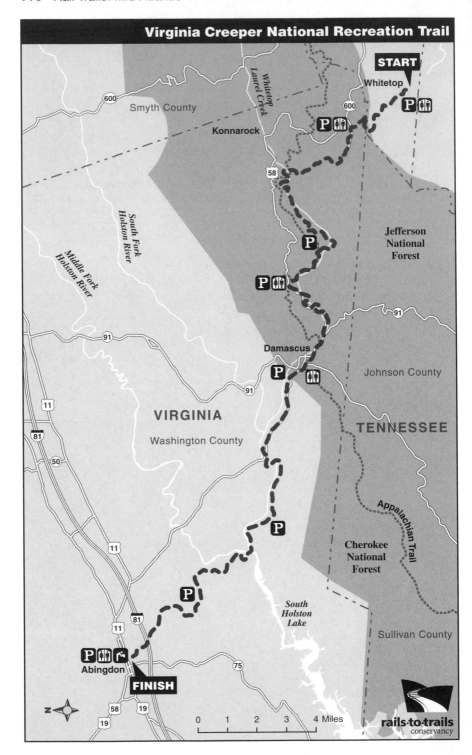

Virginia Creeper National Recreation Trail

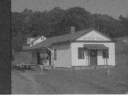

The Virginia Creeper offers scenic wonders from dense forests, open fields, and lush waterways to railroad relics and delightful small towns. Cyclists and equestrians love the length of the Creeper, and many local walkers and joggers take advantage of the pleasant opportunity for a little exercise.

The trail officially begins at the Virginia/North Carolina border, but the easiest place to start the Creeper is from the Whitetop Station trailhead. (However, to cover the entire trail, simply ride the extra mile from Whitetop to the North Carolina border before turning around to begin your voyage.)

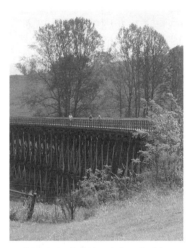

Intricate trestle bridges help make this one of Virginia's rail-trail gems.

The first 17-mile stretch to Damascus allows for numerous restroom breaks at its many trailheads, some of which are housed in restored railroad depots. This section travels through terrific scenery, from Christmas tree farms and grazing llamas to river views and deep forestland. The Appalachian Trail also weaves on and off the Creeper. After going through dense trees, you will emerge to glide over bridges high above Laurel and Green Cove creeks.

At approximately the midpoint of the Creeper, you will reach the Damascus trailhead. Before tackling the rest of the trail, consider taking a break in this sweet town. Damascus is the self-proclaimed friendliest town on the trail, and it won't take you long to see why: Its trailhead offers restrooms, a caboose-turned-information-booth, a replica train engine, and parking. Veer off the trail to find lunch stops and bike shops in town.

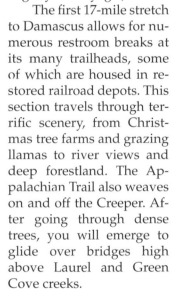

Location
Washington and Grayson counties

Endpoints
Whitetop to Abingdon

Mileage
34

Roughness Index
2

Surface
Dirt, asphalt

After your break, get ready for a little work: From Damascus to the trail's end in Abingdon, a little more effort is required. The constant downhill is exchanged for a flat grade with some gentle rises and descents. It's not strenuous, but it is a change from the first section of trail. If you are bicycling, be aware that abundant equestrian use just after Damascus can leave its mark on the trail surface and give you a bumpy ride. But don't let a few bumps get you down. They start to peter out about 7 miles before Abingdon, and some of the Creeper's most beautiful river and farmland views are still ahead.

On a ridgeline high above the South Fork Holston River, you will emerge onto a bridge offering invigorating views of South Holston Lake about 1770 feet below. Enjoy the water, cliffs, and trees while they last, because the landscape is about to change again, this time to peaceful, sprawling ranchland.

As you continue your journey toward Abingdon you will run into cattle gates across the trail. These gates mark your entrance to the Creeper's expansive grazing meadows. This tranquil farmland accompanies you for much of the remainder of the journey. About a half mile from Abingdon is a public park with restrooms, picnic areas, and a water fountain. Just across the last bridge, you will reach the endpoint.

If you are traveling to the Virginia Creeper from out of town, consider that many bike shops in Damascus and Abingdon offer bike rentals and a shuttle up to the Whitetop Station trailhead.

DIRECTIONS

To get to the Whitetop Station trailhead, follow US Hwy. 58 east from Abingdon into Grayson County. Turn right on VA Route 726 and head south toward the North Carolina border. You will see the parking area off of 726.

To get to the Abingdon trailhead, head south on Main Street (US Hwy. 11) in Abingdon and turn right onto Pecan Street. There is a large locomotive engine on display by the trailhead, which can be spotted off to the left of the parking lot.

Contact: Virginia Creeper Trail Club
           PO Box 2382
           Abingdon, VA 24212
           www.vacreepertrail.org

Washington and Old Dominion Railroad Regional Park

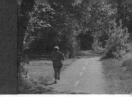

The paved W&OD Trail (as it is commonly known) is one of the region's most popular rail-trails. Used regularly by commuters headed into the Washington area, it serves as a great link between Virginia's rural and historical past and the modern city of Washington, DC.

The Washington & Old Dominion Railroad was built on the eve of the Civil War in 1858. At times both a passenger line and a freight line, the railroad eventually lost out to more efficient modes of transportation and went into disuse in 1968. In 1982, it was purchased by the Northern Virginia Parks Association, which still owns and maintains the trail today.

The trail is exceptionally well-marked, with posts indicating every half mile beginning in Shirlington, Virginia, where the trail starts in the heart of the Washington, DC-metropolitan area. From this urban setting, the trail heads though various suburban neighborhoods. Bleaumont Park (at 3.5 miles), one of many picnic areas and parks within the trail's first 10 miles, is a great rest stop, with both water and restrooms available. At 5.5 miles,

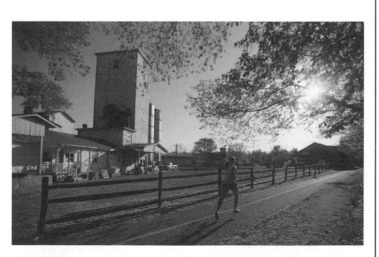

Rural Virginia farmland is found at the northern end of this trail, less than 45 miles outside of the nation's capital.

Location
Arlington, Fairfax, and Loudoun counties

Endpoints
Four Mile Run Drive in Arlington to 21st Street in Purcellville

Mileage
44.8

Roughness Index
1

Surface
Asphalt

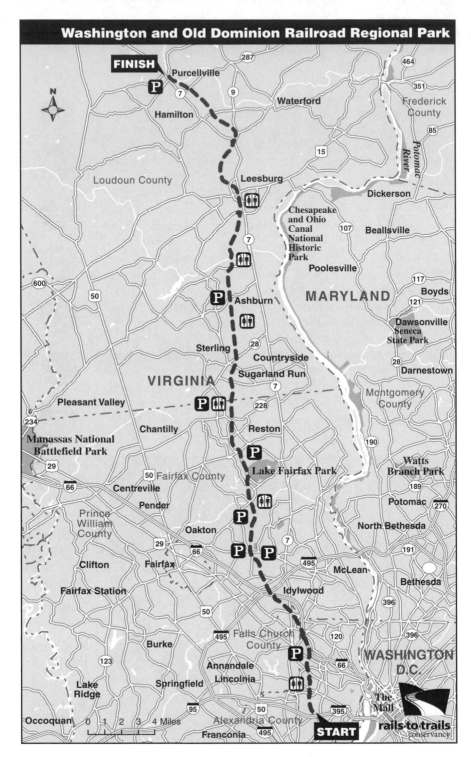

the trail provides an access point to Washington's Metrorail system by connecting to the East Falls Church Station.

As you make your way beyond the Interstate 495 beltway, at mile 9, use caution at several roads crossings, especially during rush hour. Now in Fairfax County, the trail continues through the communities of Vienna (at mile 12) and Reston (at mile 18). These suburban neighborhoods thin out a bit and the trail becomes more wooded.

The town of Herndon (at mile 20.5) is home to a wonderful trailside train depot, one of many along the trail that also provides a good rest stop. As the trail continues, it passes through Ashburn (at mile 27.5), Sterling (at mile 28), and Leesburg (at mile 34). The historical town of Leesburg has a colonial feel and is popular spot for lunch and antiquing.

The final 10 miles from Leesburg to Purcellville travel through rolling hills of classic Virginia farmland. Horses graze, corn fields flourish, and trail users can use the trip as a chance to sample Virginia wines at the many vineyards in the region. The last stop on the trail is the Purcellville Train Depot (at mile 44.8). The trail ends on a downhill ride into the town of Purcellville with a view of the Blue Ridge Mountains looming on the western horizon.

DIRECTIONS

To begin at the southern end of the W&OD Trail, take Interstate 395 to the Shirlington exit, bear right to head north, and drive to second stoplight. Turn left here on South Four Mile Run Drive. The W&OD Trail will be on the right, paralleling the road. You can park along the side of the road, but it is not advisable to leave your car overnight here.

To begin at the far northern end in Purcellville, take VA Route 7 west. Exit at VA Route 287 and turn left. Follow Route 287 until VA Business Route 7 and take a right. Turn right again on 21st Street. The Purcellville Train Depot is a quarter mile away on the right. Parking is available at the depot.

Contact: Friends of the Washington and Old Dominion Trail
21293 Smiths Switch Road
Ashburn, VA 20147
(703) 729-0596
www.wodfriends.org

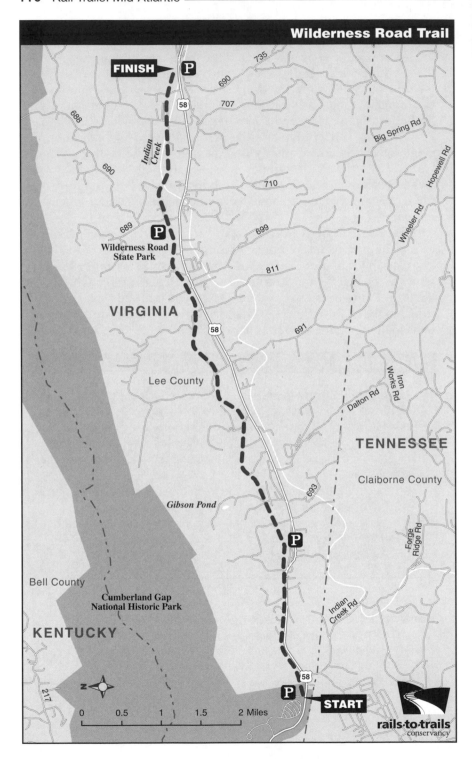

Wilderness Road Trail

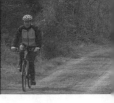

History runs deep along the Wilderness Road Trail, which roughly follows a path carved by Daniel Boone in April 1775. The path later became a route on the Louisville and Nashville Railroad before finally being converted to a rail-trail that stretches from a national historic park to a state park.

At the western trailhead in Cumberland Gap National Historic Park, the Wilderness Road Trail connects to the 1.6-mile Boone Trail, which connects to a larger trail system that continues through the Cumberland Gap.

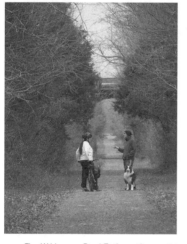

The Wilderness Road Trail provides a quiet sojourn through the country, despite its proximity to civilization.

Just beyond the trailhead in Cumberland Gap National Historic Park, you might catch a glimpse of majestic buffalo grazing in a privately owned, fenced area. The first 2 miles run right next to the four-lane US Hwy. 58. Although this sounds unpleasant, you are separated from the motorized vehicles and there is something majestic about riding through forsythia toward forest and farmland. After this stretch, the trail backs into a quiet and much more scenic area behind a veil of trees, although the path still parallels Hwy. 58 until the trail's terminus just west of Ewing.

Once it retreats from the road, the trail meanders through nearly 7 miles of picturesque farmland, complete with bright white fences and grazing cows. The route is dotted with quaint homes, barns, and silos, and the impressive Cumberland Mountain serves as a backdrop to this idyllic landscape.

Location
Lee County

Endpoints
Cumberland Gap
National Historical
Park to Ewing

Mileage
8.4

Roughness Index
2

Surface
Crushed stone

Wilderness Road State Park hosts reenactments and living history events throughout the year. The Joseph Martin House, located in the park and next to the trail, offers restrooms, a gift shop, and local history exhibits.

DIRECTIONS

To reach the westernmost trailhead in Cumberland Gap, head west from Abingdon on US Hwy. 58. Continue past the Heart of Appalachia Gazebo trailhead and paved parking lot on your right, which is about 4 miles west of Wilderness Road State Park. Continue west on Hwy. 58, and after another 2 miles, reach the trail's start point, where you'll find limited roadside parking. If you're coming from the west on Hwy. 58, the trailhead is about 1 mile east of the intersection of Hwy. 58 and US Hwy. 25.

The easternmost trailhead is also right off of Hwy. 58, at a paved parking lot about 3 miles west of Ewing. If you're heading west on Hwy. 58 from Abingdon, you'll see a sign stating that Cumberland Gap is 10 miles away. The parking area is on the north side of Hwy. 58.

Contact: Wilderness Road State Park
Route 2, Box 115
Ewing, VA 24248
(276) 445-3065
www.state.va.us/dcr/parks/wildroad.htm

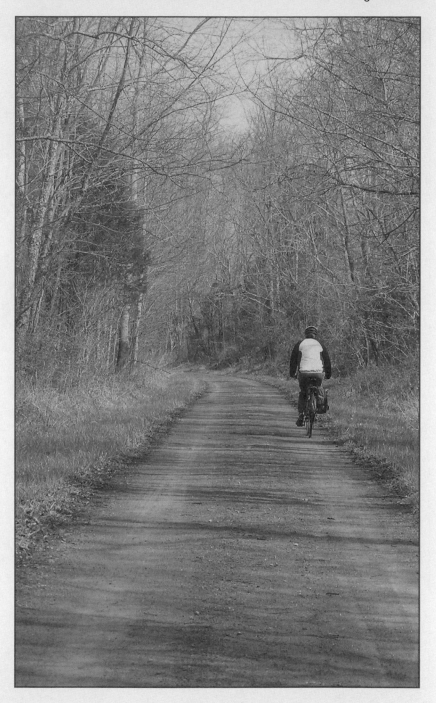

Wilderness Road Trail, Virginia

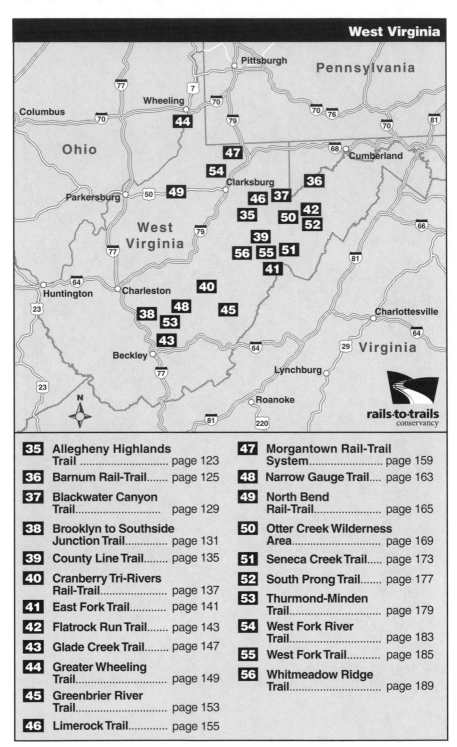

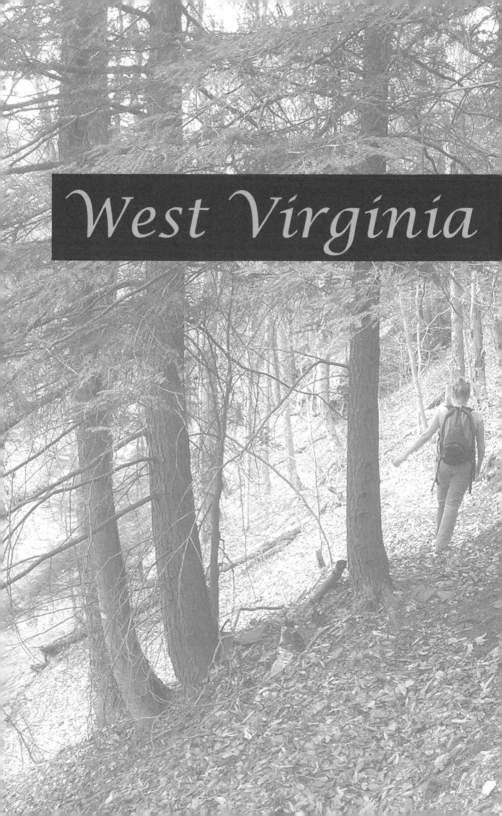

West Virginia

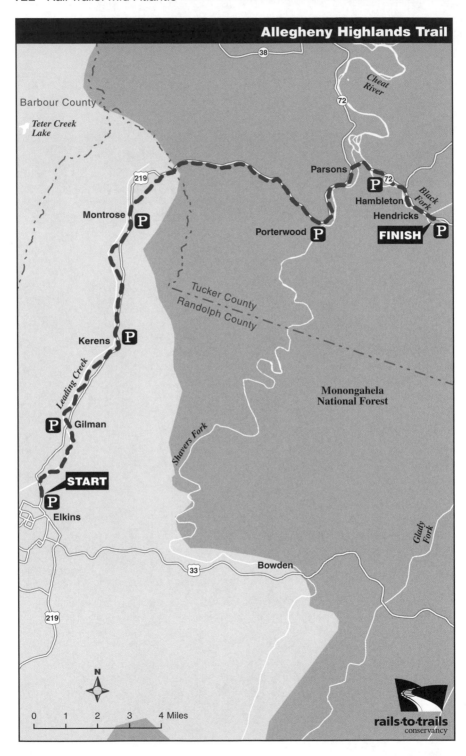

Allegheny Highlands Trail

Barbour County

Teter Creek Lake

Cheat River

38

72

219

Parsons

Montrose P

72

Hambleton

Hendricks

Porterwood P

FINISH P

Tucker County
Randolph County

Kerens P

Monongahela National Forest

Leading Creek

P Gilman

Shavers Fork

START

P Elkins

Gladys Fork

33 Bowden

219

N

0 1 2 3 4 Miles

rails·to·trails
conservancy

Allegheny Highlands Trail

The Allegheny Highlands Trail follows the original route of the West Virginia Central and Pittsburgh Railway built by Henry Gassaway Davis in 1884. For 24.5 miles, this exceptionally scenic trail provides panoramic views of the West Virginia countryside as it passes through a mountainous region with small towns and rural farmland.

From the southern Highland Park trailhead in Elkins, the trail gradually ascends for approximately 15 miles as it passes around the Pheasant and Polecat Knob mountains. The rural vistas and mountainous backgrounds provide numerous opportunities for photos. As you pass around the mountains, the trail starts to descend more steeply as it approaches the small town of Parsons.

A short, easy-to-follow, on-road section of the trail in Parsons offers the chance to grab a bite to eat at any of the several small-town restaurants. The trail continues by following US Hwy. 219 north for less than a mile, crossing the Shavers Fork and Black Fork rivers to reach

Location
Randolph and
Tucker counties

Endpoints
Elkins to Hendricks

Mileage
24.5

Roughness Index
2

Surface
Asphalt, crushed stone

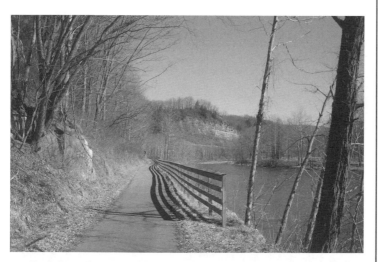

This trail runs along several waterways: Leading Creek, Shavers Fork, Black Fork, and the Cheat River—known for its impressive rapids.

the next trailhead, located just over the Black Fork River on the southern side of Hwy. 219.

The remaining 3-mile section of the trail is paved and follows the beautiful Black Fork River to the small town of Hendricks. Plans are in effect to extend the Allegheny Highlands Trail north to Mt. Storm Lake, making it approximately 44 miles in length. A path, though not the actual trail, continues along the beautifully scenic Blackwater River to the town of Thomas; however, this section is quite steep.

DIRECTIONS

From downtown Elkins, take US Hwy. 219 north to access the southernmost trailhead, Highland Park, located across from the Division of Highways District 8 Headquarters (just a mile from downtown Elkins.

The Gilman, Kerens, Montrose, and Porterwood trailheads are located mid-trail, and each include parking facilities.

Continue following US Hwy. 219 north to the northern trailhead located at the intersection of Main and 3rd streets in Hendricks.

Contact: Highlands Trail Foundation
PO Box 2862
Elkins, WV 26241
(304) 636-4519
www.highlandstrail.org

Barnum Rail-Trail

Nestled in a northern valley of West Virginia, the Barnum Rail-Trail follows the North Branch of the Potomac River through the superb scenery of the Upper Potomac region. If you plan to explore this out-and-back trail by bike, a mountain bike is the best choice for tackling the packed ballast surface.

The trail begins in the very small community of Barnum, just north of Randolph Jennings Lake in Mineral County. The trailhead (the only access point for this route) is very pleasant, with ample parking, restroom facilities, and a small park overlooking the Potomac River that offers access to incredible fishing.

Exercise caution for the first mile; the trail is open to vehicular traffic, though you probably won't encounter too many cars at this remote location. Beyond the large parking area and a closed gate, the remaining 3 miles are strictly non-motorized.

After the gate, the trail heads into the open and offers stunning views of the vibrant Potomac. Lush hillsides rise on either side of the river, and the trail hugs

Location
Mineral County

Endpoints
Barnum Road

Mileage
4

Roughness Index
2

Surface
Ballast, dirt, grass

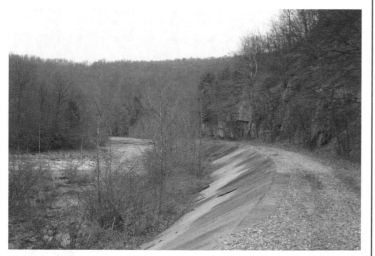

The path of the Barnum Rail-Trail is characterized by the flow of the North Branch of the Potomac River, as was the railroad itself.

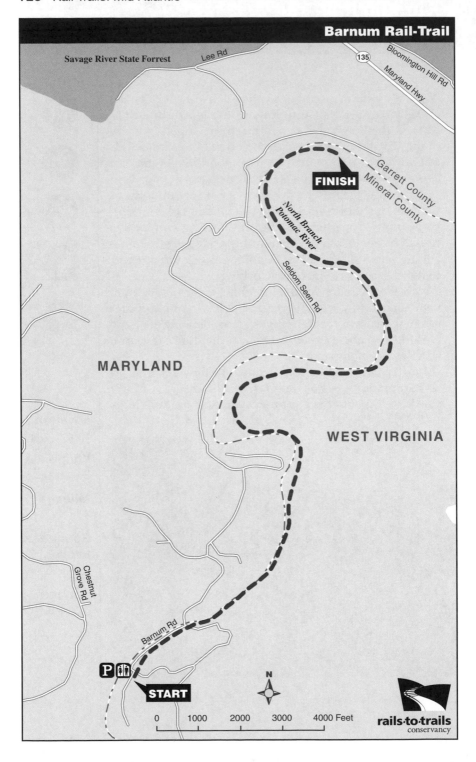

Barnum Rail-Trail

Savage River State Forrest

Lee Rd

135

Bloomington Hill Rd

Maryland Hwy

Garrett County

Mineral County

FINISH

North Branch
Potomac River

Seldom Seen Rd

MARYLAND

WEST VIRGINIA

Chestnut
Grove Rd

Barnum Rd

P

START

N

0   1000   2000   3000   4000 Feet

rails·to·trails
conservancy

the west slope while the water churns and flows immediately to your left for the next 2 miles.

The trail then enters a densely wooded area—a landscape it maintains to its northern endpoint about a mile ahead. You can hear the active rapids only a few hundred feet away at any given time. Though there is no official signage marking the end of the trail, it becomes apparent where the corridor is no longer maintained. At this point, simply turn around and enjoy the ride or walk back.

DIRECTIONS

To access the trailhead for this out-and-back trail, take US Hwy. 220 south from Keyser and then head west on US Hwy. 50. After 7 miles, take a right on WV Route 42 and then bear right onto WV Route 46. Once in Cross, take a left on Barnum Road and follow it to the end. The trail will be on the right.

Contact: Mineral County Parks and Recreation
150 Armstrong Street
Keyser, WV 26726
(304) 788-5732
www.mineralcountywv.com/index.asp

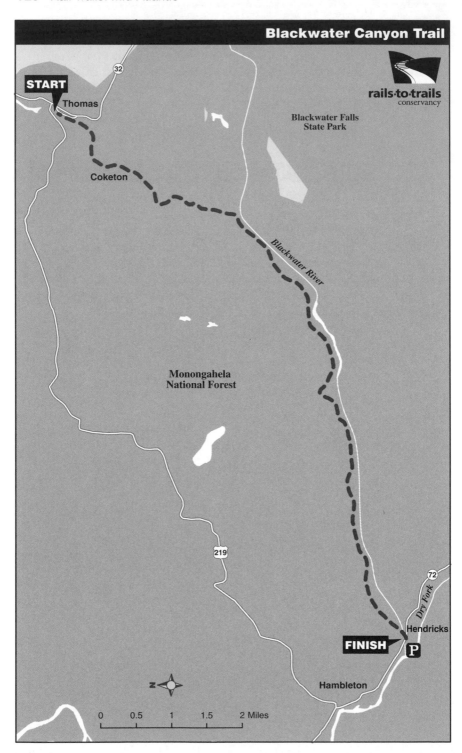

Blackwater Canyon Trail

rails·to·trails
conservancy

START
Thomas

32

Coketon

Blackwater Falls
State Park

Blackwater River

Monongahela
National Forest

219

72

Dry Fork

Hendricks

FINISH
P

Hambleton

N

0   0.5   1   1.5   2 Miles

Blackwater Canyon Trail

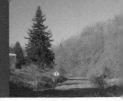

In 1888, the Blackwater Canyon Trail, located in the Monongahela National Forest, was used to haul coal and lumber through this stunning canyon. Today, remnants of this history still remain just outside of Thomas—in the form of coke ovens that line the trail along the mountainside.

The Blackwater Canyon Trail is perfect for the hiker or mountain biker in search of solitude. The relatively straight trail is beautiful, with mountains lining both sides of the canyon, and the roaring of the Blackwater River providing a soothing soundtrack. Better views of the river, including scenic waterfalls, are available during late fall, winter, and early spring, when the trees don't have as many leaves.

It is best to follow this trail from Thomas to Hendricks, as there is considerable climb in the other direction. As you travel along the Blackwater Canyon Trail, you may happen upon one of several endangered species, including the West Virginia flying squirrel, Indiana bat, or the Cheat Mountain salamander. The habitat

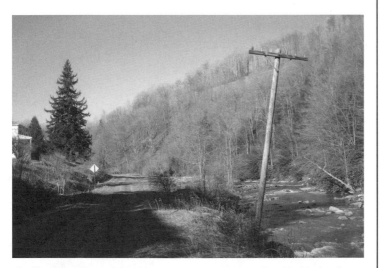

Everything in this part of the Monongahela National Forest is affected by the water that runs through the mountains.

Location
Tucker County

Endpoints
Thomas to
Hendricks

Mileage
10.3

**Roughness
Index**
3

Surface
Gravel, dirt

surrounding the trail is vital to the survival of these species, so it is important to stay on the trail. In Hendricks, it is also possible to pick up the Allegheny Highlands Trail (page 123) and Limerock Trail (page 155).

Although this beautiful trail is open to the public, a local logging company is interested in converting it into a private logging road. The Friends of the Blackwater Canyon, a local trail group, is negotiating with the Forest Service and other parties to prevent the loss of this valuable and historical resource.

DIRECTIONS

In Thomas, head south on WV Route 32 (Spruce Street). Turn right onto Douglas Road, which crosses the trail. Turn left off Douglas Road onto the trail (you can drive on this portion) to reach the trailhead approximately a mile down the road. The trailhead, where there is space for parking, is marked by a Forest Service gate. There is space there for parking.

In Hendricks, take Route 72 east through town and turn right on Second Street. The trailhead is on the right. Look for the gazebo and parking at the trailhead.

Contact: USDA Forest Service
Carol Rucker
PO Box 368
Parsons, WV 26287
(304) 478-3251
www.fs.fed.us/r9/mnf/index.shtml

Brooklyn to Southside Junction Trail

A s it weaves past long-abandoned mining towns such as Red Ash and Rush Run, the Brooklyn to Southside Junction Trail tells the unique story of "King Coal" and Appalachia. Once an important transportation corridor used to haul coal from the remote New River Gorge, this recycled railroad corridor now brings new life into the area as a tourist attraction.

Never more than 100 yards from the New River, this trail provides users with an up-close look at the natural beauty found within and along the New River Gorge National River. A forest of large oak trees, rhododendron, and evergreens envelope you as the trail meanders along the bank of the river. One of the most popular among the area's many trails, this trail is particularly attractive to mountain bikers who enjoy the rough riding provided by exposed railroad ties along its route.

Beginning at the Brooklyn trailhead, head south along the New River. Listen for the exuberant screams of whitewater rafters on the water, one of the finest whitewater rivers in the eastern US. Active railroad tracks at Southside Junction signal the temporary end of the trail.

Location
Fayette County

Endpoints
Brooklyn to
Southside Junction

Mileage
5.8

Roughness Index
2

Surface
Gravel, dirt, ballast

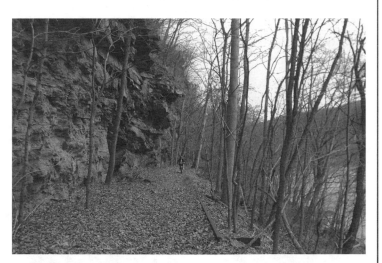

Rock bluffs along the New River make for an adventurous time on the Brooklyn to Southside Junction Trail.

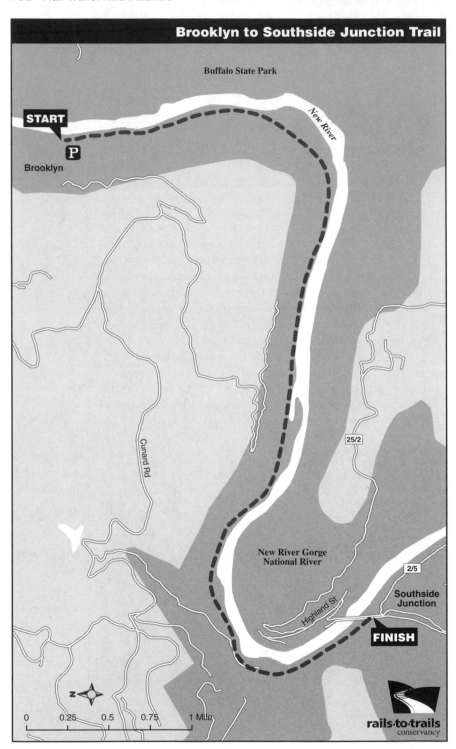

Brooklyn to Southside Junction Trail

Buffalo State Park

New River

START

P

Brooklyn

Cunard Rd

25/2

New River Gorge
National River

2/5

Highland St

Southside
Junction

FINISH

N

0   0.25   0.5   0.75   1 Mile

rails·to·trails
conservancy

While the trail extends past these tracks to a trailhead at Southside Junction, a legal (and safe) crossing here is currently not available. According to the National Park Service, negotiations are underway, but in the interim, please respect this private property and keep clear of the tracks.

DIRECTIONS

To reach the Brooklyn trailhead from Beckley, take US Route 19 north to Fayetteville. Take State Route 16 south through Fayetteville and turn left onto Gatewood Road. Turn left at the Cunard turnoff and follow signs to Cunard River Access. Once you reach the river-access area, continue 1 mile up the gravel road to the Brooklyn trailhead, where parking is available.

The Southside Junction end is not recommended as a start for the trail—the active rail line perpendicular to the trail often blocks access to the trailhead, making crossing hazardous.

Contact: New River Gorge National River
PO Box 246
Glen Jean, WV 25846
(304) 465-0508
www.nps.gov/neri/ssj_trail.htm

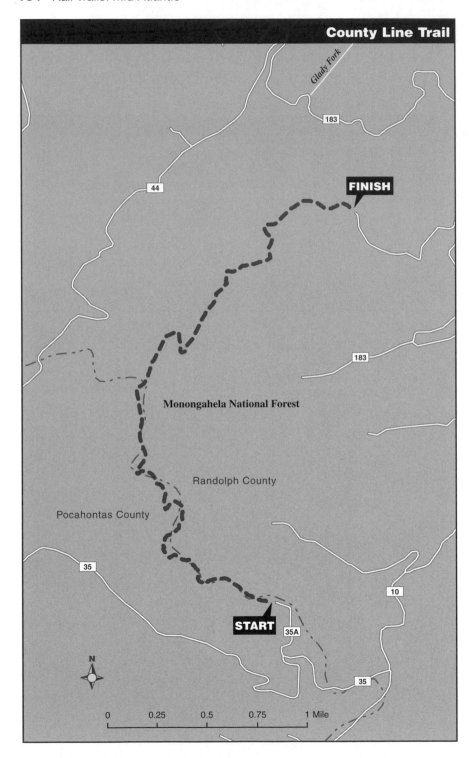

County Line Trail

The County Line Trail is a short, less-traveled alternative to the neighboring 21.7-mile West Fork Trail (page 185). The trail travels 4 miles along the border of Randolph and Pocahontas counties, hence its name, and follows the ridgeline of the Little Beech Mountain through hardwood forest in Monongahela National Forest. This area is home to impressive stands of oak trees, a slight change from the usual Monongahela setting of rhododendrons, pine trees, and ferns.

A large, green, metal gas pump sits off Forest Service Road 35A, marking the start of the County Line Trail, which is well-marked with the national forest's standard blue blazes, as well as wood arrow signs.

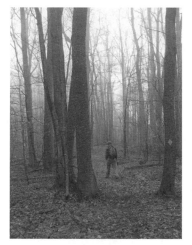

The aptly named County Line Trail splits Randolph and Pocahontas counties in the Monongahela National Forest.

Almost 3 miles in, you will make a short ascent to the top of the ridge. After another mile, you will enter a clearing for yet another gas well. The service road for this well doubles as the last leg of the trail. Follow it to reach the end of the County Line Trail, where you can either turn back around or connect to the Beulah Trail, which takes you north for another 3.3 miles.

Location
Randolph and Pocahontas counties

Endpoints
Forest Service Road 35 to the Beulah Trail

Mileage
4

Roughness Index
2

Surface
Dirt

DIRECTIONS

To get to the start point (it's not possible to drive to the endpoint) from Elkins, take US Hwy. 33/WV Route 55 east toward Bowden. About 4 miles after you travel through Bowden, turn right onto County Road 27. Once you reach the town of Glady, turn left onto County Road 22 and then take a quick right onto County Road 22-2, which turns into Forest Service Road 44 around the High Falls Trail. A little more than 7 miles from Glady, you will reach Forest Service Road 35. Follow it to Forest Service Road 35A, which ends at a gas well site. At the far end, there is a blocked road. Take this road (on foot) 40 feet to the trailhead of the County Line Trail. Parking is plentiful around the gas well.

Contact: Monongahela National Forest
200 Sycamore Street
Elkins, WV 26241
(304) 636-1800
www.fs.fed.us/r9/mnf/index.shtml

Cranberry Tri-Rivers Rail-Trail

The Cranberry Tri-Rivers Rail-Trail, also called the Cranberry Rail-Trail, is named for the Cranberry, Cherry, and Gauley rivers it travels along or across. It begins in downtown Richwood, immediately behind the visitors center, which is housed in the old passenger and freight railway depot. For the first 6 miles of this trail, you travel through town and adjacent to residents' yards. Don't be deterred by the occasional litter-strewn yard or dog that gives chase: The trail here parallels the beautiful Cherry River and is well worth the trip for the view.

Shortly after the trail crosses WV Route 55 in Holcomb, it enters Monongahela National Forest. Here, the route—now a more dedicated trail—becomes much easier to follow, with no road crossings or private property abutting it, and only the roar of the rushing water to keep you company. A beautiful waterfall on the right is visible from the conveniently located viewing platform.

After you cross the Cranberry River, the trail takes you through the curving, 640-foot Sarah's Tunnel, which is pitch dark at its center. One mile beyond the tunnel, you arrive at the trail's end. There are plans to

Location
Nicholas and
Webster counties

Endpoints
Richwood to
Allingdale

Mileage
16

**Roughness
Index**
2

Surface
Dirt, gravel

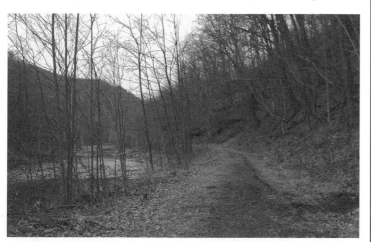

This trail features 16 miles of West Virginia wilderness adjacent to the Cherry and Gauley rivers.

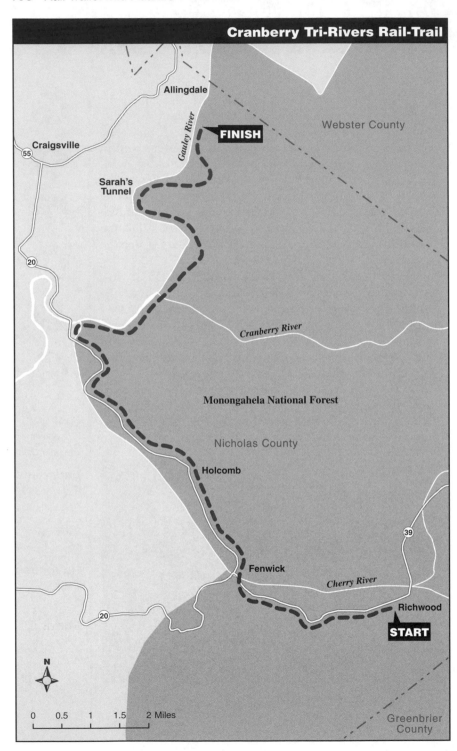

Cranberry Tri-Rivers Rail-Trail

Allingdale

Webster County

Craigsville
55

Gauley River

FINISH

Sarah's Tunnel

20

Cranberry River

Monongahela National Forest

Nicholas County

Holcomb

39

Fenwick

Cherry River

20

Richwood

START

N

0   0.5   1   1.5   2 Miles

Greenbrier County

extend the trail another 10 miles into the forest, but until that happens, please adhere to the no trespassing signs. For a longer visit, cabins are located next to the trail once you enter Monongahela National Forest. As with most trails in West Virginia, the Cranberry Tri-Rivers Rail-Trail is breathtakingly beautiful. However, the surface can be a difficult due to protruding tree roots and rocks; be prepared for thick, sticky mud just after the winter thaw.

DIRECTIONS

To reach the Richwood Trailhead, from the only traffic light in Richwood, take WV Route 39 south (downhill) and stop at the old railway depot. The trail is the gravel/dirt path behind the depot.

The Holcomb Trailhead is the recommended starting point for this trip through Monongahela National Forest. The Cranberry Tri-Rivers Rail-Trail crosses WV Route 55 on the east side of the Cherry River (if you are coming from Richwood, look for the trail before the bridge over the river). You can park at the trail entrance on the north side of the road.

Contact: Four Seasons Outfitters
190 Route 39/55 Marlington Road
Richwood, WV 26261
(304) 846-2862
www.fourseasonsoutfitter.com

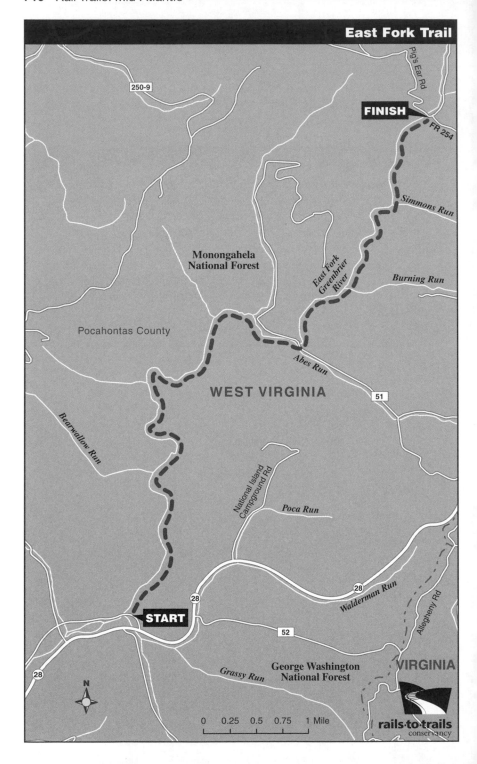

East Fork Trail

The scenic East Fork Trail follows the East Fork of the Greenbrier River through hemlock stands and pine plantations and past many small waterfalls, extending 8 miles from the Island Campground in Bartow to Pig's Ear Road (Forest Service Road 254). During the winter thaw and spring rains, this is a very wet and muddy trail, with stream crossings at mile 2.5 and near mile 6. You can avoid the first crossing by staying on the east side of the stream and looking for the trail blazes again within 300 yards.

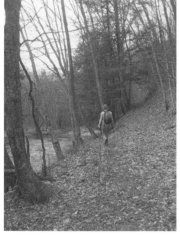

The East Fork Trail follows the path of a river, which occasionally makes for a wet walk during the winter thaw.

Anglers, rafters, and others have overnight options along the trail. In addition to the small campground at the trail's start, there are more campsites near mile 5, where the trail crosses Forest Service Road 51.

The final section of the trail leaves the banks of the Greenbrier River and follows a gradual uphill climb to Pig's Ear Road. The East Fork Trail is a treat at any time of year, but if you hit the trail during berry season, be sure to look around for tasty, wild serviceberries, also called mountain blueberries, which can be found along the entire corridor.

Location
Pocahontas County

Endpoints
Island Campground in Monongahela National Forest to Forest Service Road 254

Mileage
8

Roughness Index
2

Surface
Dirt

DIRECTIONS

From Durbin, take US Hwy. 250 east. After you pass Bartow, the highway merges with WV Route 28. Stay on Route 28, and about 6 miles from Bartow you will see signs for Island Campground, where the trail begins in the middle of the campgrounds, just off the road.

If the campsites are full and there is nowhere to park, continue going northeast on Route 28 another 5 miles to Forest Service Road 112. Follow this for about 2 miles until it forks with Forest Service Road 254. Take 254 to the end, where there is a gate marking the beginning of private property. The trail begins to the left of this gate; parking is available on the side of the road.

Contact: Monongahela National Forest
200 Sycamore Street
Elkins, WV 26241
(304) 636-1800
www.fs.fed.us/r9/mnf/

Flatrock Run Trail

West Virginia's fifth highest point, Mt. Porte Crayon, boasts dense hardwood forests, spectacular views, and a scenic hike up the Flatrock Run Trail (also known as Forest Service Trail #519). The trail is almost entirely in the Monongahela National Forest and follows one of the old logging railroad grades found all over this mountain. The hike to the majestic 4770-foot peak is strenuous, but the views from the top are well worth the effort.

The trail begins in the remote Red Creek Valley, a starting point for a great number of other wilderness trails. You will find the trailhead—the trail's only access point—located on private property off of Lanesville Road. Hikers are allowed access here through an agreement between the Forest Service and the landowner.

For its first mile, the Flatrock Run Trail makes a gradual ascent through private farmland until it meets the national forest boundary. After 3 miles and several switchbacks, you will be well above the valley floor, where the trail crosses Flatrock Run Creek. There is

Location
Tucker County

Endpoints
Red Creek Valley to
Mt. Porte Crayon

Mileage
5.5

**Roughness
Index**
3

Surface
Dirt

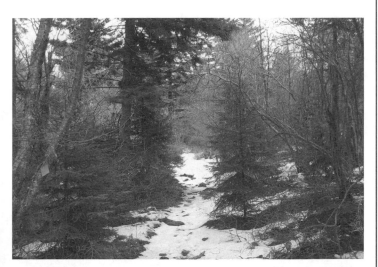

A gradual ascent and several switchbacks through a pine forest take you to a 4770-foot peak.

143

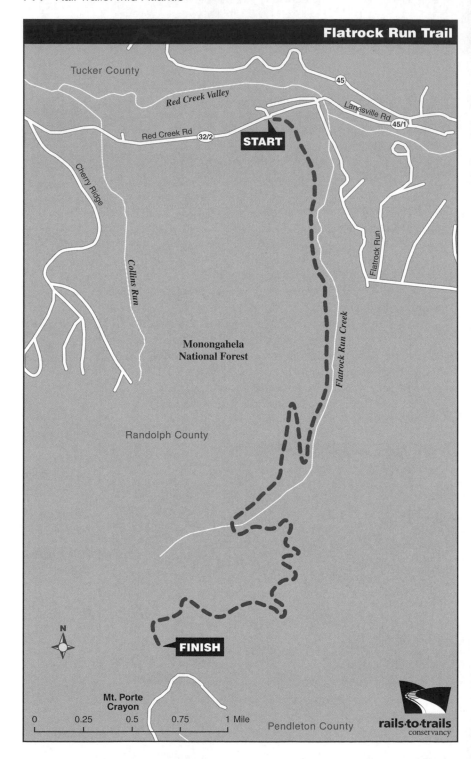

no bridge here, so use caution, especially during snow runoff in the spring. The creek, which you will follow for the entire journey, offers wonderful cascading waterfalls throughout the trail.

The last 2 miles of the Flatrock Run Trail are strenuous but rewarding. At the summit of Mt. Porte Crayon, you can pick up the Bears Nest Trail that connects to the South Prong Trail (page 177) or simply soak up the gorgeous Appalachian landscape before heading downhill for the return trip.

DIRECTIONS

From Elkins, take US Hwy. 33 east to Harmon and merge left onto WV Route 32. Travel 3.75 miles and take a right on Bonner Mountain Road. After approximately 4 miles, there will be a driveway on the right with a large barn and stable set back on top of a hill. Go up the driveway and look for the blue diamond blaze that marks the trailhead at the back of the property.

Contact: Monongahela National Forest
200 Sycamore Street
Elkins, WV 26241
(304) 636-1800
www.fs.fed.us/r9/mnf/index.shtml

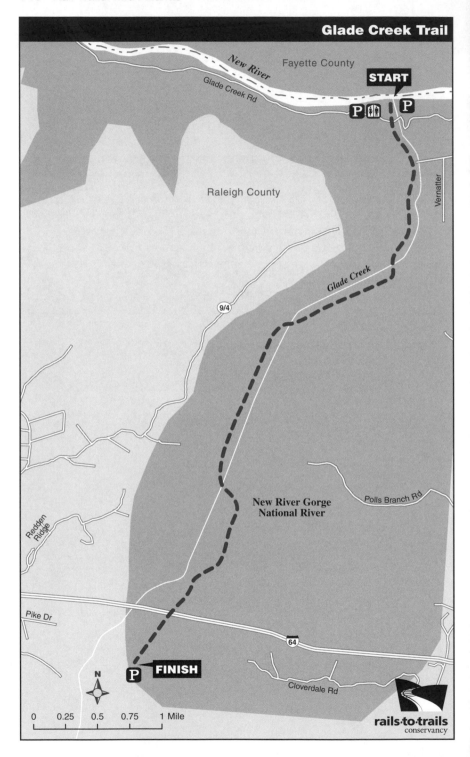

Glade Creek Trail

Fayette County

New River

Glade Creek Rd

START

Vernatter

Raleigh County

Glade Creek

9/4

Polls Branch Rd

New River Gorge
National River

Redden Ridge

Pike Dr

64

P FINISH

Cloverdale Rd

N

0   0.25   0.5   0.75   1 Mile

rails·to·trails
conservancy

Glade Creek Trail

Situated in the heart of West Virginia's pristine New River Gorge National River, the Glade Creek Trail (out-and-back only) has something for everyone. Once a narrow gauge railroad corridor used to haul coal from remote mines within New River Gorge, Glade Creek Trail is now a popular destination for hiking, swimming, fishing, camping, and kayaking.

Start your trip at the trailhead located near the confluence of Glade Creek and the New River. Here you will find several well-maintained campsites, picnic tables, and restrooms. The trailhead is also home to a popular swimming hole that is a great place to cool off after a hot summer hike.

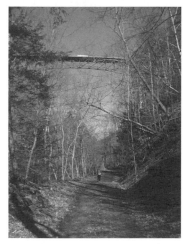

This trail passes beneath one of several towering single-arch bridges, one of which is popular with base jumpers.

Once on the trail, you can enjoy the beautiful scenery and picturesque waterfalls provided by Glade Creek, as it rushes past on its way to the New River. Be sure to bring your fishing pole, as the lower section of Glade Creek is an official catch-and-release trout stream. As the trail meanders along the banks of the creek, keep an eye out for native wildlife and the occasional adventurous kayaker attempting to navigate the creek's swift rapids.

The Glade Creek Trail has a moderate grade, but the first half can be difficult to hike, as the path is slightly narrow and frequently strewn with large rocks and tree branches. Once you cross the trail's lone bridge, found around the 3-mile mark, the trail becomes wider and better maintained. If you're looking for a challenge, hit the more strenuous Kates Falls Trail located about 1 mile before the end of Glade Creek Trail.

Location
Raleigh County

Endpoint
Glade Creek

Mileage
6

Roughness Index
2

Surface
Gravel, dirt

DIRECTIONS

From Beckley, follow US Hwy. 19 north toward Oak Hill and then drive north on WV Route 41 toward Prince. Turn right onto Glade Creek Road, just before the bridge in Prince. Follow the gravel road for 7 miles to the Glade Creek Trailhead.

Contact: New River Gorge National River
PO Box 246
Glen Jean, WV 25846
(304) 465-0508
www.nps.gov/neri/glade_creek.htm

Greater Wheeling Trail

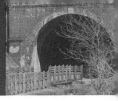

The Greater Wheeling Trail starts at Pike Island Locks and Dam, and provides an urban escape and an opportunity to soak up local history and modern industry in this historic city.

The entire trail is flat and paved, and beautiful signs along the route provide a self-guided tour of Wheeling's historical past. At its core is the Ohio River, the powerful and one-time lifeblood of the city's manufacturing industry. This trail travels under the massive bridge spanning the river and connecting Wheeling with Ohio and the rest of the west. Barges still go up and down the river, and with good timing and patience you can watch one progress through the series of locks.

A couple miles from the start and just before the Wheeling Convention Center is a colorful playground. If you are traveling with children, stop in to play on the monkey bars, or simply sit back and enjoy some quality people-watching from one of the trail's many benches or from one of the eateries nearby. If you pick the right place, you will be rewarded with a splendid view of the river, wildlife, and many trail users.

Location
Ohio County

Endpoints
Pike Island Locks and Dam to 48th and Water streets

Mileage
14

Roughness Index
1

Surface
Asphalt

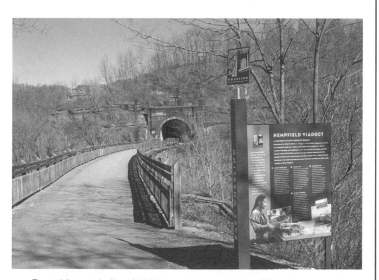

This trail features the Hempfield Viaduct and a tunnel built in 1904.

149

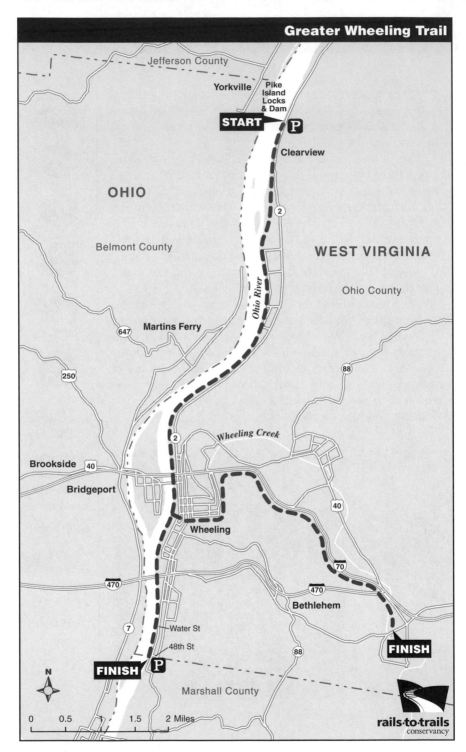

The trail is in constant use by people of all ages. Multiple residential neighborhoods (as well as a Wal-Mart) border the trail, so you will likely see locals walking or riding to purchase groceries and supplies. Students, particularly elementary school children on their way to school, use the trail, too.

DIRECTIONS

To get to the starting point from downtown Wheeling, travel north on River Road and look for Pike Island Locks and Dam on the left. The parking lot is in front of the dam. The endpoint is located at the intersection of 48th Street and Water Street in downtown Wheeling.

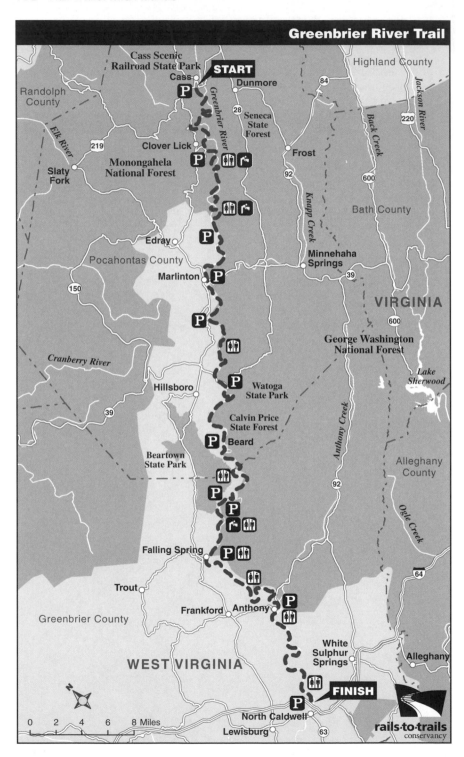

Greenbrier River Trail

W est Virginia's beautiful Greenbrier River Trail is one of America's premier rail-trails—popular with bicyclists, hikers, walkers, and cross-country skiers. Most of the trail runs along the gorgeous Greenbrier River and passes through picturesque West Virginia countryside and local townships as it winds through the river valley. There is no doubt that you will see many forms of interesting wildlife along this wonderful trail.

Today, the trail is operated and maintained by West Virginia State Parks, but it was originally built for use by one of the many West Virginia railroads that serviced the once prospering local timber industry. Now the trail is for recreational use, with overnight campsites and many restroom and water facilities scattered along its route. For the last 20 years, the trail has hosted the popular annual Great Greenbrier River Race, which consists of a canoeing, biking, and running leg.

Even though the mile posts start at the southern terminus of the trail, it's best to start your trip on the slightly uphill grade at the northern terminus at Cass Scenic Railroad State Park and follow the river downstream. The first town you will pass is Clover Lick, a lovely little

Location
Greenbrier and
Pocahontas
counties

Endpoints
Cass Scenic Railroad State Park to
North Caldwell

Mileage
77

Roughness Index
2

Surface
Gravel

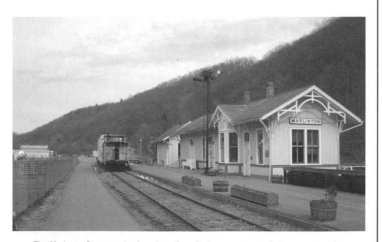

The Marlinton Depot on the Greenbrier River Trail serves as a trailside museum with exhibits on the former railroad.

Appalachian town with rustic remnants of the old railroad depot that once served the booming logging industry.

Beyond the Clover Lick trailhead, the trail proceeds south, winding 20 miles downstream through some of the most scenic and remote wilderness landscapes in West Virginia. This section ends at the only large town you will encounter along the trail, Marlinton, which hosts some great lunch spots and bed-and-breakfasts. You can find a trailside information center in Marlinton's old train station near mile 55. As you proceed south from Marlinton, you will cross the river twice before reaching the halfway point at Beard.

Beyond Beard, at mile marker 31, is one of the trails' two spectacular tunnels: the 402-foot-long Droop Mountain Tunnel, built in 1900. The other is Sharps Tunnel, just beyond mile point 65. Work began on the impressive, 511-foot-long structure in 1899. These tunnels are a reminder: One of the great things about the Greenbrier is the opportunity to see remnants of the old railroad, including the many whistleposts and historical mile markers.

Continuing south, beyond Anthony (at mile 15), the trail crosses two former railroad bridges and eventually reaches its southern terminus at North Caldwell (mile post 3). This trailhead is located just outside Lewisburg, which has a variety of shops, restaurants, and lodging establishments.

DIRECTIONS

To reach the northern trailhead at Cass, take US Hwy. 219 to WV Route 66 east, or take WV Route 28 to Route 66 west and look for trailhead at Cass Scenic Railroad State Park along Route 66.

To reach the southern trailhead at North Caldwell, take Interstate 64 east and take exit 175 to US Hwy. 60 west. Take this 2.7 miles to WV Route 38/Stone House Road. If you're coming from Interstate 64 west, take exit 169 to US Hwy. 219 north, and then take this a half mile to WV Route 30/Brush Road. From here, drive another half mile to Route 38/Stone House Road.

Contact: Monongahela National Forest Headquarters
200 Sycamore Street
Elkins, WV 26241
(304) 636-1800
www.greenbrierrivertrail.com

Limerock Trail

The Limerock Trail is pure West Virginia: From Forest Service Road 18, the 4-mile rail-trail passes through rhododendron forests and along rocky cliffs and rushing streams. You begin with the sound of the rapids from Tub Run, and they quietly disappear as you head west down the ridge toward Hendricks.

There are several places on the trail where you will have to traverse a stream. When the water level is low, it's possible to do this by rock-hopping; otherwise, your feet will get wet. After about 1.5 miles, you will reach Big Run, where the blue blazes marking the path become more sporadic; however, the trail is still easy to follow. After Big Run, you will come to Flat Rock Run. Departing briefly from the trail and following this creek downhill will bring you to a 20-foot waterfall.

The trail ends at the Blackwater Canyon Trail (page 129). To avoid the Limerock Trail's uphill return hike, you can follow the Blackwater Canyon about 5 miles north to Coketon or 2 miles south to Hendricks.

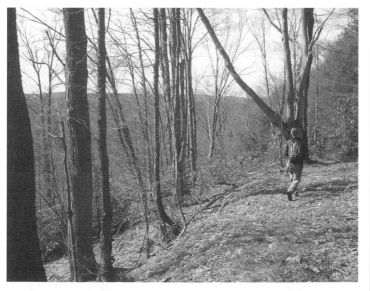

A high cliff face along the Limerock Trail provides amazing views of the Blackwater River and surrounding hillsides.

Location
Tucker County

Endpoints
Forest Service Road 18 to Blackwater Canyon Trail in Monongahela National Forest

Mileage
4

Roughness Index
2

Surface
Dirt

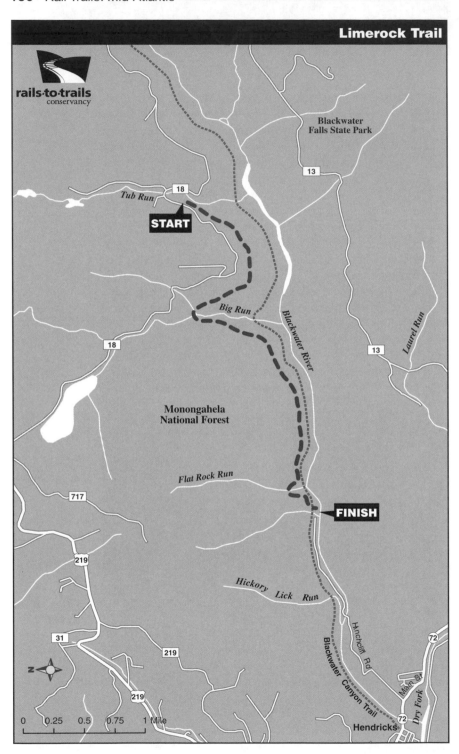

Limerock Trail

rails·to·trails
conservancy

Blackwater
Falls State Park

13

Tub Run

18

START

Big Run

Blackwater River

18

13

Laurel Run

Monongahela
National Forest

Flat Rock Run

717

FINISH

219

Hickory Lick Run

31

Hinchcliff Rd.

72

219

Blackwater Canyon Trail

Main St.

Dry Fork

N

219

0   0.25   0.5   0.75   1 Mile

72

Hendricks

DIRECTIONS

From Elkins, take US Hwy. 219 north toward Parsons. About 10 miles after you pass Parsons, you will see a sign on the right for Forest Service Road 18. Turn right here and then take the next left, which is actually the continuation of Forest Service Road 18 (there is no sign indicating this). You will need a four-wheel-drive vehicle to reach the trail on this road, as it is not paved and is very rutted, with at least one stream crossing. After about 3.5 miles, you will see a sign for the Limerock Trail on your right. You may park on the side of the road.

For a longer hike, you can take US Hwy. 219 toward Parsons and then take WV Route 72 to Hendricks. On Route 72, you will see to your right the Allegheny Highlands Trail trailhead. Park in this lot, located near the Blackwater River on your right, and take the Allegheny Highlands Trail (page 123) across Route 72 to the Blackwater Canyon Trail. This trail will meet Limerock about 2 miles north of Hendricks.

Contact: Monongahela National Forest
200 Sycamore Street
Elkins, WV 26241
(304) 636-1800
www.fs.fed.us/r9/mnf/index.shtml

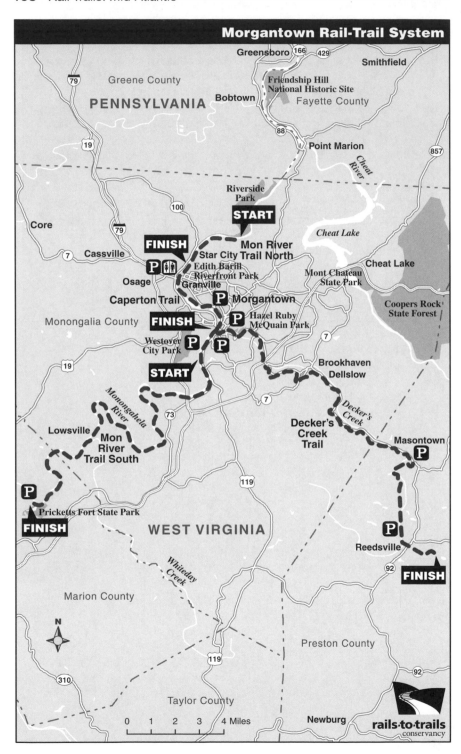

Morgantown Rail-Trail System

Greensboro 166 429

Smithfield

Greene County

79

PENNSYLVANIA

Bobtown

Friendship Hill
National Historic Site

Fayette County

19

Point Marion

857

88

Cheat River

Riverside Park

100

START

Core

Cheat Lake

79

Cassville

FINISH

P

Mon River
Star City Trail North

Cheat Lake

7

Osage

P

Edith Barill
Riverfront Park

Mont Chateau
State Park

Granville

Caperton Trail

P

Morgantown

Coopers Rock
State Forest

Monongalia County

FINISH

P

Hazel Ruby
McQuain Park

Westover
City Park

P

P

7

START

Brookhaven
Dellslow

7

73

Decker's Creek

Monongahela River

Decker's
Creek
Trail

Masontown

Lowsville

Mon
River
Trail South

P

119

P

Reedsville

P

Pricketts Fort State Park

92

FINISH

FINISH

WEST VIRGINIA

Whiteday Creek

Marion County

N

Preston County

310

119

92

Taylor County

0 1 2 3 4 Miles

Newburg

rails·to·trails
conservancy

Morgantown Rail-Trail System

Morgantown is known as the home of the University of West Virginia, the inspiration for a Joni Mitchell song, and the birthplace of Don Knotts. But soon the Morgantown area will also be known for its wonderful trail system.

The nexus of this 45-mile trail system is Hazel Ruby McQuain Park in downtown Morgantown. Located adjacent to a restored railway station, the park is a vibrant hub of local activity, with a steady stream of walkers, runners, skaters, and cyclists. The rail-trail that runs through the park—stretching 6.5 miles to the north and 19.5 miles to the south—hugs the Monongahela River, one of a few American rivers that flows north. The "Mon" eventually arrives in Pittsburgh, where it joins the Allegheny River to form the Ohio River.

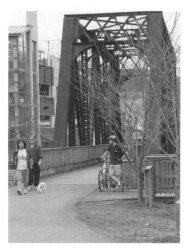

Homes and businesses are accessible around the Morgantown Rail-Trail System.

This stretch of trail, which follows a former CSX rail line, comprises three segments with three different names. The middle section, the Caperton Trail, named after a former West Virginia governor, is a paved 5.5-mile route within the city of Morgantown. This trail parallels the river past retail businesses, the university, industrial areas, and the back decks of eateries that cater to trail users.

The Mon River Trail North is a crushed-stone trail that starts a half mile north of Star City, a small town north of Morgantown. It ends abruptly after 2.7 miles, when you reach a bridge that has not been restored. When fully developed, this section of trail will extend 4

Location
Marion, Monongalia, and Preston counties

Endpoints
Morgantown

Mileage
45

Roughness Index
1

Surface
Asphalt, crushed stone

more miles to the Pennsylvania state line, where it will one day connect with trails near Point Marion, Pennsylvania.

The Mon River Trail South begins where the paved trail becomes crushed stone at the southern edge of Morgantown. From there, it meanders for 17.8 miles to Pricketts Fort State Park. The Mon South lazily winds along the many twists and turns of the Monongahela, and it is a delight to travel through this wooded riparian landscape.

The Decker's Creek Trail is the gem of the system. Beginning at the confluence of the Monongahela River and Decker's Creek at Hazel Ruby McQuain Park, the trail stretches 19 miles to the southeast, gaining 1000 feet as it climbs out of the Monongahela River valley. The first 2.5 miles of the Decker's Creek Trail are paved, passing through an unremarkable urban landscape in Morgantown. But all that changes after the trail turns to crushed stone and passes under Interstate 68. As the ascent begins, you enter a rural landscape distinguished by hemlock, rhododendron, and a smattering of residences. But the most memorable feature of this landscape is Decker's Creek itself. Because of the steady grade, the trail passes a series of dramatic rapids and waterfalls as the creek noisily rushes headlong toward the Monongahela.

As you continue the climb, Dave's Snack Shack is a welcome respite at mile 9. Proprietor Dave Lewis offers cold drinks, a comfortable seat in the shade, and a generous helping of local lore. This is not to be missed. As the trail approaches its endpoint near Reedsville, the grade flattens and the woods give way to wetland areas that feature cattails and red-winged blackbirds.

For those not accustomed to rail-trails that require hard pedaling, you can start on the Reedsville end and enjoy a pleasant ride downhill into Morgantown.

DIRECTIONS

To reach the Hazel Ruby McQuain Park from Interstate 68 west, take exit 7 and go 0.3 mile. Turn right on Count Road 857 south and go 1 mile. Turn left on US Hwy. 119 (Mileground Road/North Willey Street). Go 3 miles and turn left as Hwy. 119 becomes High Street. Go 1 mile and turn right on Moreland Street. Hazel Ruby McQuain Park is in less than a quarter mile.

To reach Edith Barill Riverfront Park, take WV Route 7 north from downtown Morgantown (Don Knotts Blvd./University Blvd./Beechhurst Ave./Monongahela Blvd.) to Star City.

To reach Pricketts Fort State Park from Interstate 79, take exit 139 north of Fairmont and follow signs to the park.

To reach the Reedsville trailhead from Morgantown, take Route 7 southeast toward Reedsville for about 17 miles. In Reedsville, continue straight on Route 92. Go 0.8 mile to the trailhead.

Contact: www.morgantown.com/trails.htm

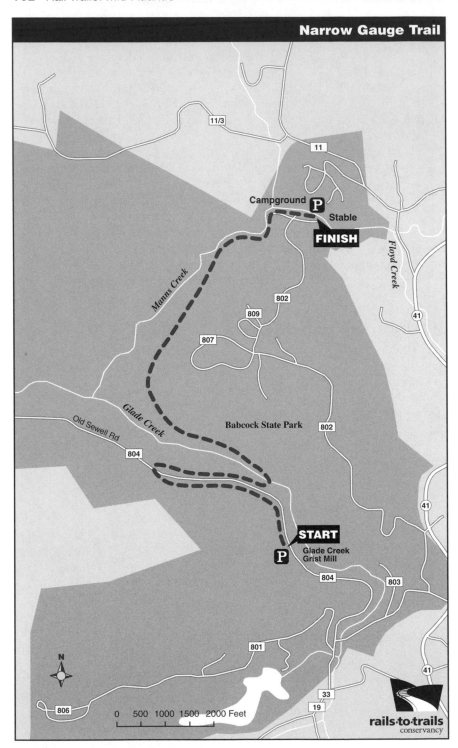

Narrow Gauge Trail

11/3

11

Campground   P
Stable
FINISH

Manns Creek

Floyd Creek

802

809

807

41

Glade Creek

Old Sewell Rd

Babcock State Park

804

802

41

START

P   Glade Creek
Grist Mill

804

803

41

801

N

806

0 500 1000 1500 2000 Feet

33
19

rails-to-trails
conservancy

Narrow Gauge Trail

The Narrow Gauge Trail in Babcock State Park follows the gentle grade of what was the Manns Creek Railway, which connected Clifftop to Sewel until it closed in 1956. The trail is breathtaking, but be forewarned: If you are not an accomplished mountain biker, you should consider it a hiking trail. The name rings true, as the trail is very narrow, tends to sit less than a foot away from a cliff over a shallow creek, and is occasionally blocked by boulders, forcing you to scale the cliff a bit on trail detours.

Before heading out on the trail, be sure to take a moment to enjoy the Glade Creek Grist Mill, arguably the most photographed site in West Virginia. Built in 1976 from parts of older mills found all over West Virginia, its design is based on the 1890 Stoney Creek Grist Mill. The mill is fully operational and offers park guests freshly ground buckwheat, whole-wheat flour, and cornmeal during the summer months when it is open.

From Cabin #13, which you can rent from Babcock State Park, it is almost a mile downhill to the official start of the Narrow Gauge Trail. Along the trail, Manns

Location
Fayette County

Endpoints
Old Sewell Road to Babcock State Park

Mileage
3

Roughness Index
2

Surface
Gravel, dirt

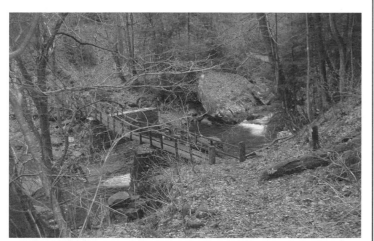

Truly a "narrow" trail, the Narrow Gauge Trail makes for an exciting hike, but mountain bikers should be experienced if they want to tackle this trail.

Creek provides the soundtrack as you travel through a beautiful example of a typical West Virginia mountain forest, with secondary hardwood and pine trees peppered among rhododendron bushes. The trail ends between the Babcock State Park campgrounds and the stables.

DIRECTIONS

To reach both ends of the trail, from US Hwy. 19, take the US Hwy. 60 exit and head east for 10 miles to WV Route 41, heading south. The trail can be accessed from the campground, which is 2 miles south of Hwy. 60 at Clifftop (the trail begins on the service road between the campgrounds and the stables). This entrance is open only in the summer.

The trail also can be accessed from the main park entrance, a little farther south on WV Route 41, behind Cabin #13. Follow the signs to Cabin #13 from the entrance: Go behind the Glade Creek Grist Mill and follow that road (Old Sewell Road) past the cabins to the official start of the trail at the fork of the creek. The trail is downhill from the cabins to the campground.

Contact: Babcock State Park
HC 35, Box 150
Clifftop, WV 25831
(304) 438-3004
www.babcocksp.com

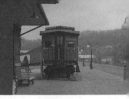

For a weekend getaway filled with small-town charm, wildlife, and beautiful natural scenery, there is no better place than the North Bend Rail-Trail.

The North Bend Rail-Trail is a scenic excursion along part of the 5500-mile, coast-to-coast American Discovery Trail. Stretching nearly 70 miles from Interstate 77 near Parkersburg to Wolf Summit, the trail travels through an impressive 13 tunnels, crosses 36 bridges, and passes through an assortment of state, county, and local parks.

Though it is easily accessible from interstates 77 and 79 and runs parallel to US Route 50, the trail passes through wild and natural areas. You will find an abundance of wildlife, including deer and beaver, and the farmland surrounding the small, rural communities that grew up along the railroad corridor provide prime bird-watching. The North Bend Rail-Trail's many points of interest and history include the former Stage Coach Inn in Pennsboro, a marble factory, hand-blown glass factories, outlet stores, arts-and-crafts markets, fairs and festivals, sites of train robberies, and legends of tunnel ghosts.

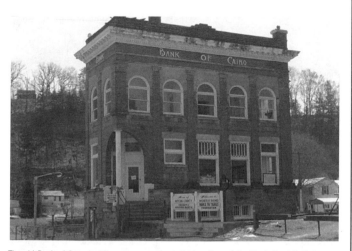

The old Bank of Cairo building serves as the trailside office of the North Bend Rails to Trails Foundation.

Location
Harrison, Doddridge, Ritchie, and Woods counties

Endpoints
Parkersburg to Wolf Summit

Mileage
69.1

Roughness Index
3

Surface
Crushed stone, ballast, cinder, grass, gravel, dirt

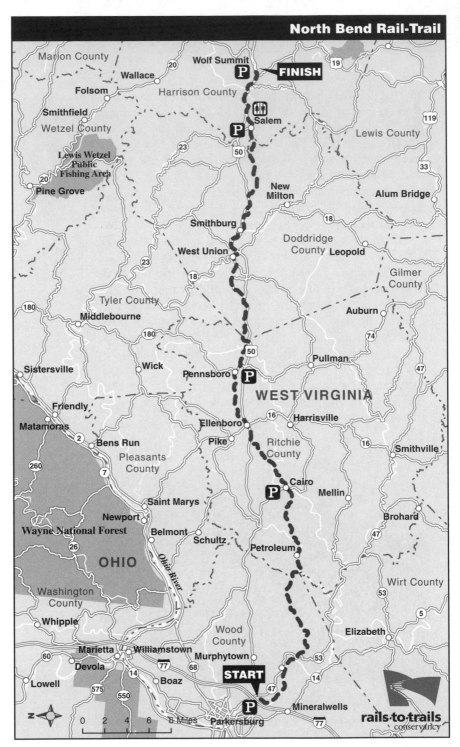

In the tumultuous years before the Civil War and the creation of the state of West Virginia, the rail corridor was constructed by the Baltimore and Ohio Railroad between 1853 and 1857. Thirteen of the railroad's original tunnels remain. The number 10 tunnel, west of Ellenboro, is 337 feet long and is a "raw" or natural tunnel, meaning it was bored through solid rock. Many of the tunnels are quite long and require a flashlight or headlamp to safely navigate them.

The true gem of this trail is the stunning natural scenery. Beyond the spectacular bridges and tunnels, the undisturbed beauty you are exploring makes you feel more like the explorers Lewis and Clarke than a 21st century mountain biker or hiker. While safety is always a concern while cycling, remember to keep your head up, too, or you may miss the numerous opportunities for wildlife encounters—especially the bountiful deer.

You'll also encounter other trail users, particularly near the many quaint towns along the trail that have wholly embraced the rail-trail, building eateries that will satisfy even the hungriest of bikers and hikers. Towns such as Cairo, Pennsboro, and Salem have all had restaurants pop up next to the trail. The locals are happy to share a story of the old rail line, and the staffs welcome even the sweatiest of customers.

DIRECTIONS

To reach Parkersburg trailhead, take Interstate 77 to the Staunton Ave. exit and turn east on WV Route 47. Take the first right turn (about 0.2 mile from interstate) on Old WV Route 47. Continue about 0.7 mile and turn right on Happy Valley Road. Travel approximately 0.4 mile until you see a large house on the left. Immediately after the stone wall (Millers Landing) is the North Bend Rail-Trail. Park on the gravel section opposite the trailhead.

To begin at Wolf Summit, take US Hwy. 50 to the Wolf Summit exit north. The trail crosses the exit.

Contact: North Bend Rail-Trail
Route 1, Box 221
Cairo, WV 26337
(304) 643-2931
www.wvparks.com/northbendrailtrail

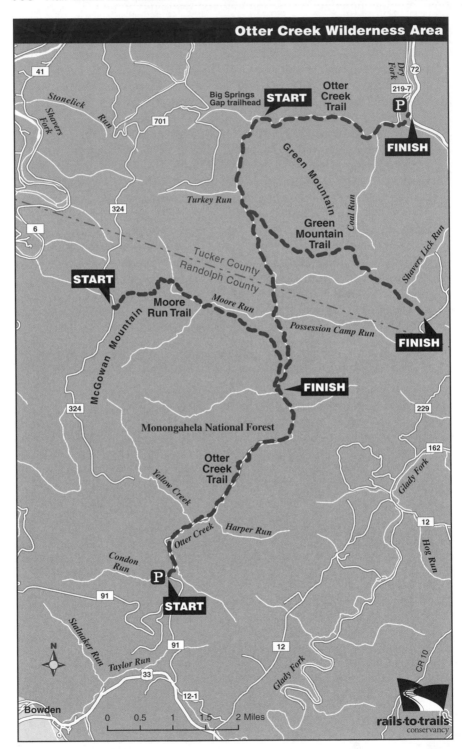

Otter Creek Wilderness Area

Otter Creek Wilderness Area

The Otter Creek Wilderness Area, located 10 miles northeast of Elkins, is a hiker's paradise. Federally protected since 1975, the area prohibits the use of all vehicles, including bikes, so hikers alone have access to the Otter Creek drainage area, surrounding mountains, and 20,000 acres of undisturbed forest.

The extensive system features dozens of trails throughout the wilderness area, including three rail-trails, which are historical remnants of the area's once booming logging industry. Attempts have been made to keep the area primitive, so no bridges or other human structures can be found. Be prepared to get wet while crossing any number of streams.

Though a cairn marks each trail intersection, the trails themselves are not well-marked. Be sure to pick up a map of the entire system at the National Forest Service office in Elkins.

Location
Randolph County

Endpoints
Monongahela
National Forest

Mileage
19

Roughness Index
3

Surface
Dirt

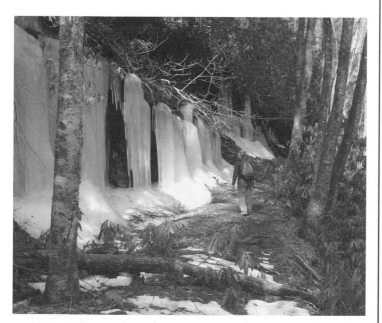

As water leeches from the hillsides in the Otter Creek Wilderness Area, frigid mountain temperatures create stalactites of ice.

169

OTTER CREEK TRAIL

You might not guess that the Otter Creek Trail is a rail-trail. Built on a turn-of-the century timber-logging corridor, the trail follows Otter Creek for 11 very rugged miles. Running from one end of the Monongahela National Forest's Otter Creek Wilderness Area to the other, the Otter Creek Trail serves as a spine to the wilderness area's extensive trail system.

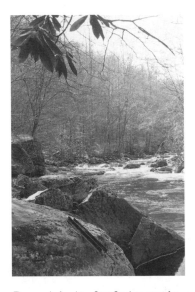

The sound of rushing Otter Creek is never far away on this rail-trail.

The Otter Creek Trail offers spectacular views and a moderate to challenging hike. You will find yourself following large rock outcrops and peering through trees at roaring waterfalls. There are a number of stream crossings along its path and, depending on the season, some are quite significant, with fast, rushing water. With the exception of a very long, suspended footbridge over the Dry Fork tributary of the Cheat River toward the end of the trail, there are no bridges to aid your stream crossings.

Like all of the trails in the Otter Creek Wilderness Area, attention has been given to keeping this trail very primitive. There are no signs or blazes. However, confusing sections are marked with stone cairns. This rail-trail is not for the faint of heart, but it is worth the hike if you are up for a challenge.

DIRECTIONS

From Elkins to the southern trailhead, take US Hwy. 33 to reach Forest Service Road 91 (Alpena Gap) and turn left. Follow the road until you see signs for the trailhead.

From Parsons to the northern trailhead, take WV Route 72 south. Look for trailhead signs along the Dry Fork River; the turn will be on your right.

GREEN MOUNTAIN TRAIL

This scenic hike accesses some of the most remote areas of Otter Creek Wilderness. Stretching 4 miles, this trail offers stunning views of the remote West Virginia backcountry and has less traffic than other trails in the region due to its difficult accessibility. The Green Mountain Trail is great for either an overnight backpacking trip or a long and challenging dayhike.

Although the trail itself is 4 miles long, there is some considerable hiking to get to the start of the trail. The trail can best be accessed by hiking in from the Big Spring Gap trailhead or either of the Otter Creek trailheads.

The trail starts by climbing steeply out of the Otter Creek valley, which provides breathtaking views of the surrounding area. It levels out after about 2 miles and follows a high mountain plateau before reaching the junction with the Possession Camp Trail after 2.7 miles. The trail concludes with a 1.3-mile ascent through thickly wooded brush at the top of Green Mountain. The end of the trail is marked by a cairn indicating the start of the Shavers Mountain Trail.

DIRECTIONS

To reach Big Spring Gap trailhead, from Parsons, take 1st Street north to Billings Ave. and turn right onto Billings. Billings turns into County Road 219. Turn right on Forest Service Road 701 and follow the signs to the trailhead, which will be on the left.

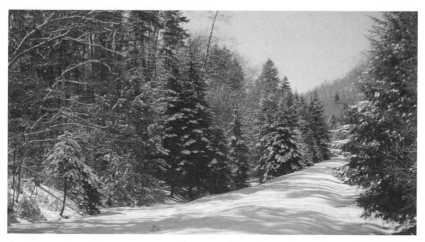

The old berm of the railroad bed is still visible through a blanket of snow on the Green Mountain Trail.

MOORE RUN TRAIL

The trailhead for the 4-mile Moore Run Trail is marked simply with a posted sign along Forest Service Road 324. You may need to look closely for the trail itself, as the overgrowth of rhododendron around the trailhead can obscure it. However, once you find the trail near the creek bed, it is easy to follow the entire way.

The trail begins by following Moore Run (a creek) for about 2 miles. You will pass through two high mountain meadows and cross several small streams. After 2 miles, as the trail starts to steadily descend down McGowan Mountain toward Otter Creek, you will be treated to the sights and sounds of this remote region. Listen for the rushing rapids of Otter Creek far below. The view over the valley and of the mountains in the distance is breathtaking. Also watch for various forms of wildlife, including small mammals and birds that are found throughout this entire wilderness area.

The trail terminates at the valley floor, where it meets another rail-trail, the Otter Creek Trail, and the Possession Camp Trail. To reach both of these trails, you must cross the rather wide Otter Creek, so hike up your pant legs and plunge in—carefully!—if you plan to continue your trail adventure on the opposite shore.

DIRECTIONS

From Parsons, take County Road 219 south, and turn left on County Road 39 in the town of Porterwood. Continue to the town of Pheasant Run and turn left on Forest Service Road 828. Turn right on Forest Service Road 701 and then turn right on Forest Service Road 324, heading south. The trailhead, though hard to spot, is on the left.

Contact: Monongahela National Forest Headquarters
200 Sycamore Street
Elkins, WV 26241
(304) 636-1800
www.fs.fed.us/r9/mnf/index.shtml

Seneca Creek Trail

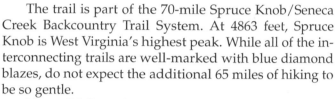

Located in the Seneca Rocks National Recreation Area of the Monongahela National Forest—a hotspot for mountain biking and rock climbing—the Seneca Creek Trail is a scenic feast of streams, meadows, forest, and waterfalls. Unlike other rail-trails in the national forest, this out-and-back route shows characteristics typical of former railroad corridors: It is flat and provides a relatively steady, easy hike and is doable with a mountain bike.

The trail is part of the 70-mile Spruce Knob/Seneca Creek Backcountry Trail System. At 4863 feet, Spruce Knob is West Virginia's highest peak. While all of the interconnecting trails are well-marked with blue diamond blazes, do not expect the additional 65 miles of hiking to be so gentle.

The trail follows Seneca Creek, a fast-flowing, spring-fed mountain stream whose clean, crystal water can be heard and seen nearly everywhere along the trail. From the trailhead, you'll immediately pass through meadows

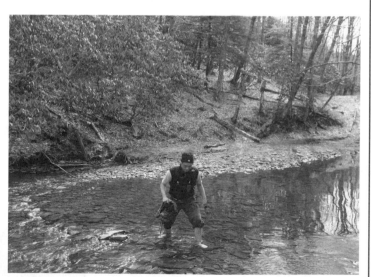

The Seneca Creek Trail mandates a stream crossing, but it's worth it for the amazing trail experience that ends at Upper Seneca Creek Falls.

Location
Pendleton County

Endpoint
Monongahela
National Forest

Mileage
5

**Roughness
Index**
3

Surface
Dirt

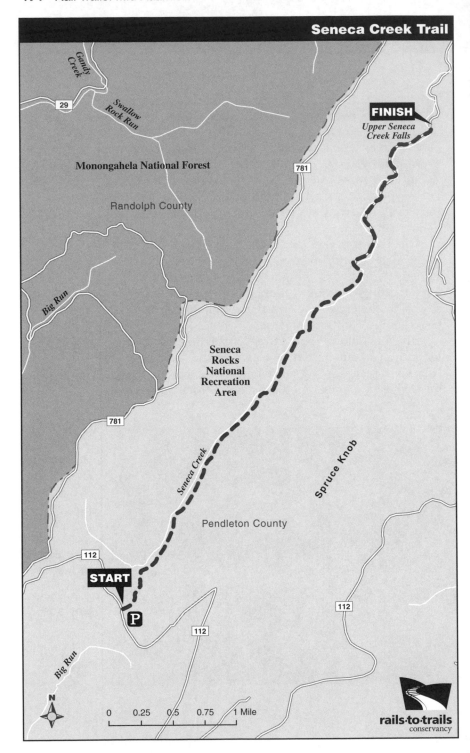

and spruce groves. A few miles in, you will encounter hardwoods. A canopy of maple, beech, birch, and cherry create a natural tunnel, offering a wide array of color in the fall and shade in the summer.

Multiple creek crossings dot this trail, and there are no footbridges, so come prepared to get your feet wet. Near the trail's end, the last—and most rewarding—creek crossing brings you to the 30-foot Upper Seneca Creek Falls. The spectacular falls are the highest on Seneca Creek and offer a dramatic finale to this trail.

DIRECTIONS

From Elkins, take US Hwy. 33 south to Briery Gap Road (County Road 33) and turn right. Follow it approximately 2.5 miles until you reach Forest Service Road 112 (this steep, narrow, gravel road is not maintained in winter) and turn right. Drive approximately 11 miles until you reach the trailhead on your right. Limited parking is available.

Contact: Monongahela National Forest Headquarters
200 Sycamore Street
Elkins, WV 26241
(304) 636-1800
www.fs.fed.us/r9/mnf/index.shtml

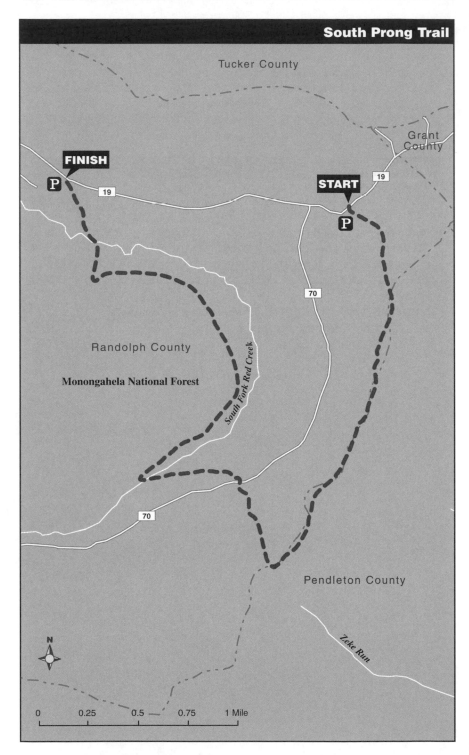

South Prong Trail

The South Prong Trail is a remote, rugged rail-trail that offers a moderate, though sometimes quite hilly, hike. There are two very distinct sections of this trail; one section is boggy, while the other is steep and forested.

Traversing the Flatrock Plains and Roaring Plains of Monongahela National Forest, this trail follows old logging corridors for part of its route. The western end follows approximately 3 miles of terraced rail beds along a flat corridor for a short while before heading uphill, or downhill, to the next terrace of rail beds, located almost vertically 15 to 25 feet below or above you.

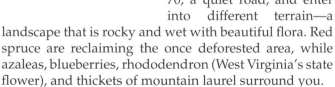

The South Prong Trail is blazed with blue diamonds, but be careful if you are starting from the eastern end. The blazes marking the turnoff points through the terraced rail beds can be easy to overlook.

The trail reaches an elevation of 4130 feet and then levels off, following the eastern continental divide. Near the midsection, you will cross Forest Service Road 70, a quiet road, and enter into different terrain—a

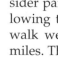
Rhododendron groves line this trail.

landscape that is rocky and wet with beautiful flora. Red spruce are reclaiming the once deforested area, while azaleas, blueberries, rhododendron (West Virginia's state flower), and thickets of mountain laurel surround you.

To turn your out-and-back trip into a loop trail, consider parking your car at the western trailhead and following the trail east. Once you've completed the hike, walk west along quiet Forest Service Road 19 for 1.5 miles. This will take you from the eastern trailhead back to the western trailhead, where you can close the loop.

Location
Randolph and Pendleton counties

Endpoint
Forest Service Road 19 in Monongahela National Forest

Mileage
5.5

Roughness Index
3

Surface
Dirt

DIRECTIONS

From Elkins, take US Hwy. 33/ WV Route 55 east to WV Route 32 and turn left, now heading north toward Cannon Valley Resort State Park. Turn right onto County Road 32 and continue until the road dead-ends into County Road 45. Turn right here and cross over Red Creek. This road turns into Forest Service Road 19, a steep, narrow, gravel road. Be careful navigating it. Go approximately 1 mile and you will see the South Prong/Boar's Nest trailheads. Turn right into small parking area. This is near the west end of the trail.

To reach the east end, continue on Forest Service Road 19 another 1.5 miles until you reach a small trailhead with parking.

Contact: Monongahela National Forest
200 Sycamore Street
Elkins, WV 26241
(304) 636-1800
www.fs.fed.us/r9/mnf/index.shtml

Thurmond-Minden Trail

With breathtaking scenery, numerous bridges, and several impressive overlooks, it is no wonder that the wide, well-maintained Thurmond-Minden Trail is one of the most popular trails in New River Gorge National River.

The trail traces the Arbuckle Branch railroad corridor along the banks of three rushing waterways from the old mining community of Minden to the historic railroad town of Thurmond. Though the Arbuckle Branch, built in 1906, was abandoned long ago, you can still see evidence of coal mining along this route.

The trail begins along scenic Arbuckle Creek and follows the raging water of this tributary to its confluence with the New River. Near the banks of the New River, be sure to stop at the overlook for an incredible view of the New River and an active railroad line. After a brief journey along the New River, the trail heads south along the quiet banks of Dunloup Creek. The trail ends at a parking lot near a popular fishing hole.

Location
Fayette County

Endpoints
Thurmond to Minden

Mileage
3.2

Roughness Index
2

Surface
Gravel, dirt

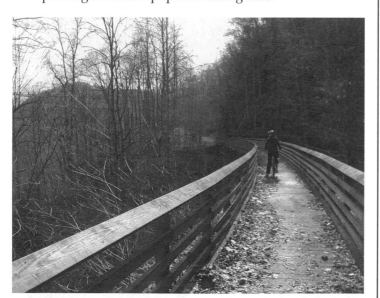

The Thurmond-Minden Trail is an impressively maintained rail-trail with beautiful views from this bridge.

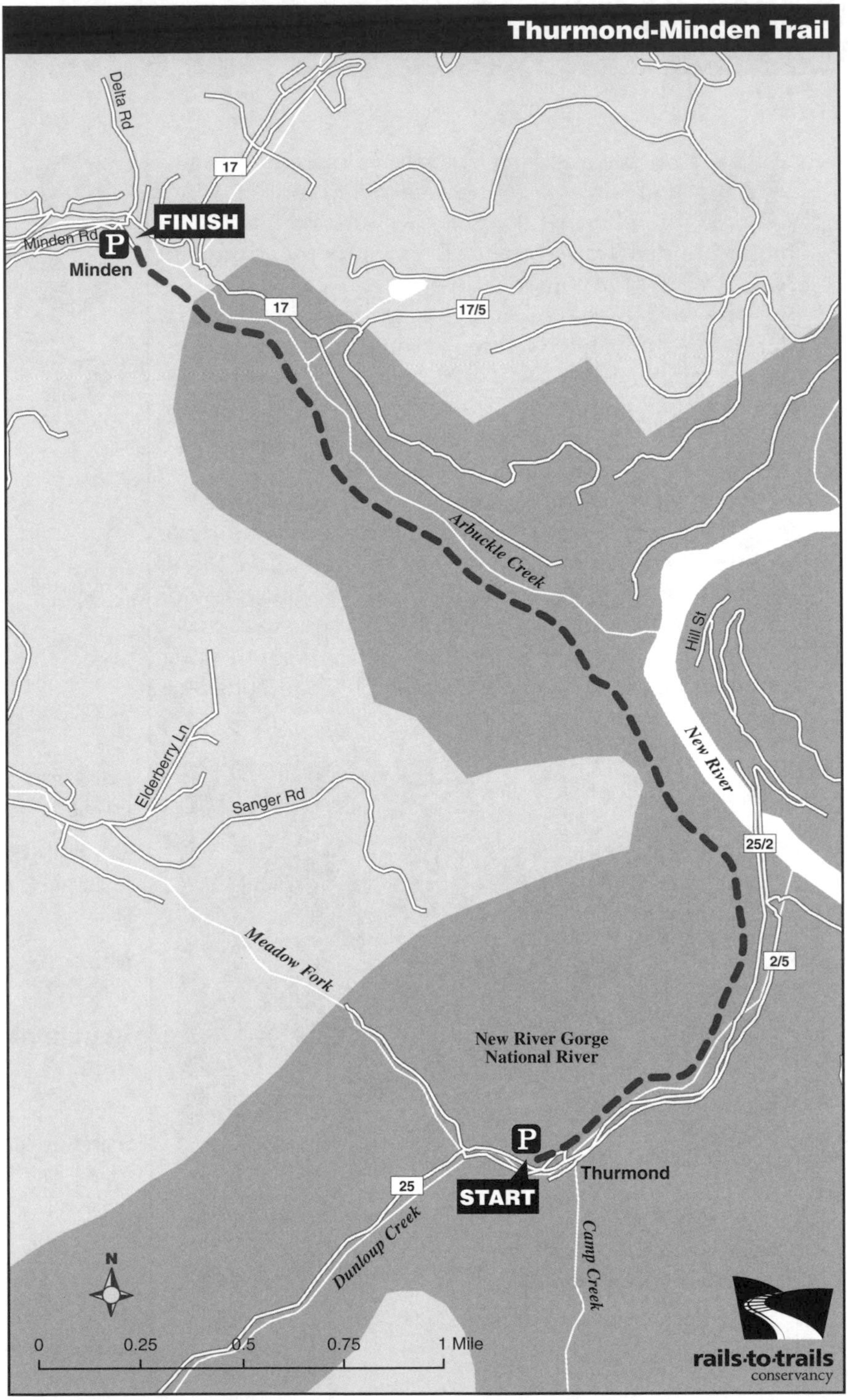

Thurmond-Minden Trail

Delta Rd

17

Minden Rd

FINISH

P

Minden

17

17/5

Arbuckle Creek

Hill St

New River

Elderberry Ln

Sanger Rd

25/2

Meadow Fork

2/5

New River Gorge
National River

P

Thurmond

25

START

Dunloup Creek

Camp Creek

N

0   0.25   0.5   0.75   1 Mile

rails·to·trails
conservancy

While the Thurmond-Minden Trail provides an excellent path for bicycling and hiking, bikers beware: A set of stairs built around the remains of a rockslide can hinder your journey if you are unable to carry your bike up and down the wooden steps.

DIRECTIONS

To access the Thurmond trailhead, head north from Beckley on US Hwy. 19. Take the Glen Jean-Thurmond exit and turn left onto WV Route 25. Go a half mile to Glen Jean, following the signs for the Thurmond-Minden Trail, located 5 miles outside of Glen Jean off Route 25.

To reach the Minden trailhead from Beckley, head north on US Route 19. Take the Oak Hill/Main Street exit and turn right onto East Main Street at the end of the ramp. Turn left at Minden Road and follow it for 2 miles. Take a right across a small bridge to the Minden trailhead.

Contact: New River Gorge National River
PO Box 246
Glen Jean, WV 25846
(304) 465-0508
www.nps.gov/neri/tm_trail.htm

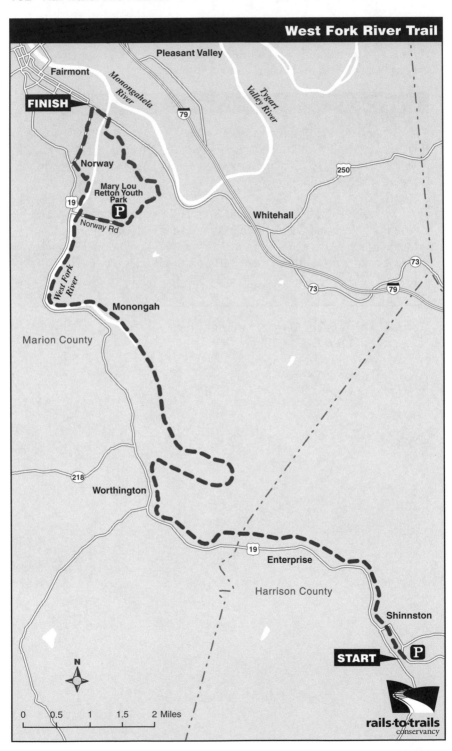

West Fork River Trail

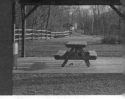

West Virginia's West Fork River Trail provides a snapshot of some of the most beautiful scenery in this region. The trail's path was once used by the far-reaching Baltimore & Ohio Railroad to deliver coal. Today's plans however, are to transport people and link this rail-trail to the American Discovery Trail.

Shortly after its start in picturesque Shinnston, the trail reaches rippling West Fork River and its cliffs and forests. Close to the Harrison and Marion county border, you will pass an historical railroad bridge that spans the river. The trail travels through some wooded passages, and then it opens up to a park where children play baseball and softball and fisherman vie for the prized catch below the dam. A few miles beyond that, you cross a railroad bridge and are returned to the wooded haven of the trail.

At the town of Norway, you have the option of going another half mile on to a stunning wooden bridge, or you can continue past the bridge to the Mary Lou Retton Youth Park, which offers recreational fields, parking, restrooms, and the West Virginia Miners' Memorial. Pay close attention for the turnoff for the park:

Location
Harrison and
Marion counties

Endpoints
Shinnston to
Fairmont

Mileage
18.3

**Roughness
Index**
2

Surface
Crushed stone,
cinder, gravel

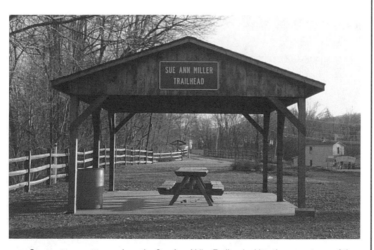

Community amenities such as the Sue Ann Miller Trailhead add to the convenience of the West Fork River Trail.

As you head toward the town of Fairmont, the turnoff is on the right. After turning off the trail, turn left to reach the park on the paved road (unmarked County Road 56/6), and then take a quick right uphill on unmarked Norway Road through the little town of Norway.

DIRECTIONS

The starting point in Shinnston is accessible from US Hwy. 19 on the southern end of town. To reach Shinnston from the Shinnston/Saltwell Road exit off Interstate 79, turn left (west) and proceed a quarter mile to the Exxon station. Turn left on Saltwell Road (WV Route 131) and follow this about 7 miles to Hwy. 19 in Shinnston. Turn right onto Hwy. 19 (Pike Street) and drive six blocks. Turn left on Mahlon Street at St. Ann's Catholic Church, before the bridge across the West Fork River. Go one block and park on the street. The trail begins under the Hwy. 19 bridge. Future plans call for a trailhead parking lot to be built along Hwy. 19.

To reach the northern terminus in Fairmont from the US Hwy. 250 exit (exit 132) off Interstate 79, go north on Hwy. 250. At the Pizza Hut, turn left and follow Mary Lou Retton Drive to Mary Lou Retton Youth Park. Park here and walk or ride to the top of the driveway. Follow signs approximately 1 mile on Norway Road to the trail. At the trail, turn left to go in the direction of Shinnston.

Contact: Marion County Park and Recreation Commission
316 Monroe Street
Fairmont, WV 26554
(304) 363-7037
www.mcparc.com/parks/westfork.htm

West Fork Trail

The West Fork Trail is a pleasant 21.7-mile trail that snakes its way through a remote mountain setting and follows the West Fork River for most of its route. The soothing rumble of the river complements the trail's serene environment. This is a great path for biking, but the surface is primarily ballast left over from the rail corridor, so leave your road bike at home.

The trail begins in the small community of Glady. Even though the trail appears to be flat, you will find yourself on a gentle decline as the trail follows the river downstream from Glady. For the first 5 miles, the trail takes a higher route above the western side of the river and pops in and out of small groves of conifers, offering great views of the surrounding hills.

The trail then levels out with the river and travels the remaining 17 miles to the town of Durbin following the river southward. Meandering through the mountains, the trail and the river make sweeping 180-degree turns through a tight valley surrounded by steep hillsides.

The West Fork River is a popular fishing spot, and you are bound to see a number of anglers along the way.

Location
Randolph County

Endpoints
Glady to Durbin

Mileage
21.7

Roughness Index
2

Surface
Crushed stone, ballast, gravel

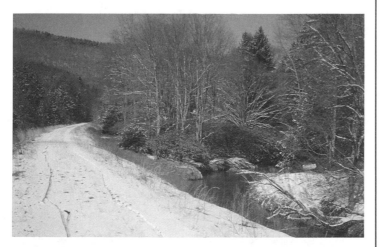

This trail curves along the West Fork River, negotiating the snug turns through the hills and valley.

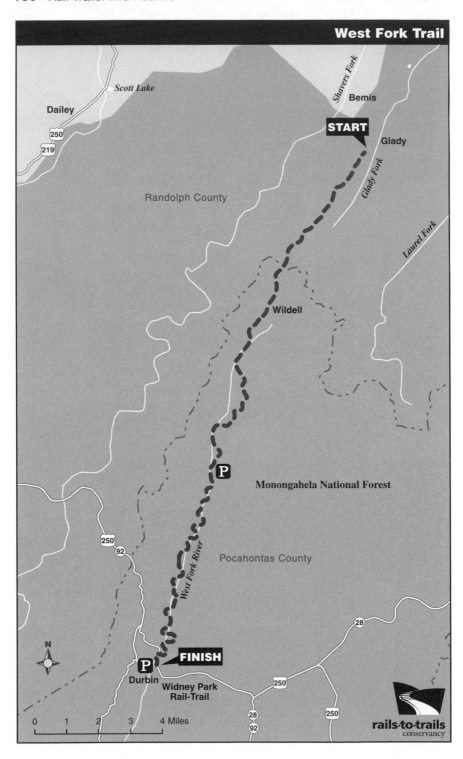

West Fork Trail

Scott Lake

Dailey

250
219

Shavers Fork

Bemis

START

Glady

Glady Fork

Randolph County

Laurel Fork

Wildell

P

Monongahela National Forest

250
92

Pocahontas County

West Fork River

28

N

28
92

250

P
Durbin

FINISH

Widney Park
Rail-Trail

250

250

0   1   2   3   4 Miles

rails·to·trails
conservancy

The trail comes to an end in the town of Durbin, a quiet Appalachian town that has wonderful little lunch spots and a nice Main Street corridor. There is a bonus half-mile rail-trail, the Widney Park Rail-Trail, which can be accessed right in downtown Durbin.

DIRECTIONS

To reach the northern trailhead from Elkins, take US Hwy. 33 east and make a right onto County Road 27 (Glady Road). Follow it for approximately 10 miles to the town of Glady. When you come to the intersection of Glady and Elliots roads, continue straight on Glady through the stop sign and follow the road for approximately a quarter mile to where it dead-ends. The trailhead will be directly in front of you.

To reach the southern trailhead from Elkins, take US Hwy. 219 south to Huttonsville. Merge onto US Hwy. 250 going south and follow it all the way to Durbin. Look for the trailhead on the left about a mile before you reach the town.

Contact: Monongahela National Forest
200 Sycamore Street
Elkins, WV 26241
(304) 636-1800
www.fs.fed.us/r9/mnf/index.shtml

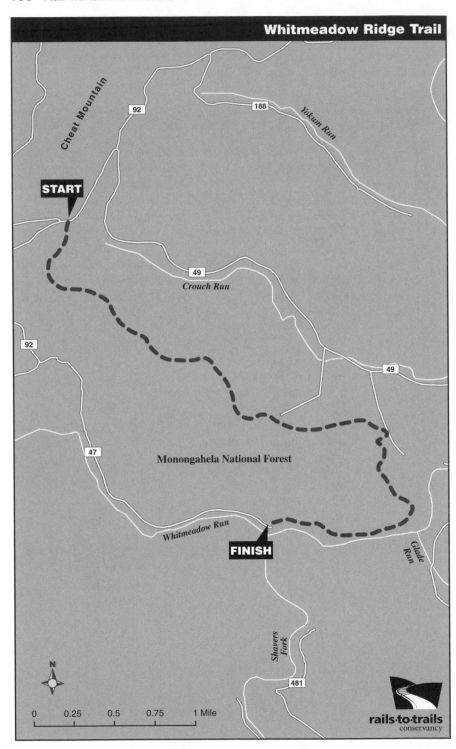

Whitmeadow Ridge Trail

Cheat Mountain

92

188

Yokum Run

START

49
Crouch Run

92

49

47

Monongahela National Forest

Whitmeadow Run

FINISH

Glade Run

Shavers Fork

481

N

0   0.25   0.5   0.75   1 Mile

rails·to·trails
conservancy

Whitmeadow Ridge Trail

Located in the heart of West Virginia, the Whitmeadow Ridge Trail is also in the center of the Monongahela National Park. Otherwise known as the Whitmeadow Hunters Access Trail (notice the bullet holes in the trail signs), this beautiful trail follows the ridgeline of Cheat Mountain 4.7 miles to Shavers Fork. It travels through a secondary forest of pines, oaks, and several different fern species.

There is about a 1000-foot descent from the beginning off Forest Service Road 92 to the end. This descent is not gradual until it reaches the old railroad bed near Shavers Fork. The trail parallels Shavers Fork through a rhododendron forest until it reaches the end, where Shavers Fork meets Whitmeadow Run. The parking area is next to a catch-and-release fishing hole that is also perfect for picnics, though there are no facilities.

The drive to the trail is also beautiful. The highway route from Elkins to Forest Service Road 92 is known as the Cheat Mountain Backway, a scenic highway that passes the site of the Cheat Mountain Summit Fort where Union Troops camped in the summer of 1861. There are now interpretive signs around the grounds to tell the story to visitors.

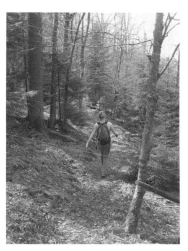

The Whitmeadow Ridge Trail offers a lovely walk through secondary pine and oak forests.

Location
Randolph County

Endpoints
Forest Service Road 92 to Shavers Fork, Monongahela National Forest

Mileage
4.7

Roughness Index
2

Surface
Dirt

DIRECTIONS

From Elkins, take US Hwy. 219 south toward Huttonsville. After you drive through Huttonsville, take US Hwy. 250/WV Route 92 south for 7 miles toward Durbin. Turn left onto Forest Service Road 92. Look for the northwest trailhead about 1.3 miles north after you cross Forest Service Road 47.

To access the southeast trailhead from Forest Service Road 92, turn right onto Forest Service Road 47 and drive to its end. Here you will find a large parking lot next to Shavers Fork. Both ends of the trail are signed.

Contact: Monongahela National Forest
200 Sycamore Street
Elkins, WV 26241
(304) 636-1800
www.fs.fed.us/r9/mnf/index.shtml

STAFF PICKS

Popular Rail-Trails

When Rails-to-Trails Conservancy staff members scoured the Mid-Atlantic for great rail-trails, these were the ones that stood out as their favorites. Short or long, city or country, these are rail-trails not to miss.

Delaware
Junction and Breakwater Trail

Maryland
Allegheny Highlands Trail Maryland

Capital Crescent Trail

Number Nine Trolly Line

Western Maryland Rail Trail

Virginia
Devils Fork Loop Trail

Huckleberry Trail

New River Trail State Park

Virginia Creeper National Recreation Trail

Washington and Old Dominion Railroad Regional Park

West Virginia
Allegheny Highlands Trail

County Line Trail

Glade Creek Trail

Greenbrier River Trail

Narrow Gauge Trail

Otter Creek Wilderness Area

For History Buffs

These rail-trails don't just challenge your body, they engage your mind. Pick up some historical facts on these trails.

Delaware
Tri-Valley Trail

Maryland
Baltimore and Annapolis Trail

MA & PA Heritage Trail

Virginia
Hanging Rock Battlefield Trail

Staunton River Battlefield Rail-Trail

Wilderness Road Trail

West Virginia
Greenbrier River Trail

ACKNOWLEDGMENTS

Each of the trails in *Rail-Trails: Mid-Atlantic* was personally visited by RTC staff. Maps, photos, and trail descriptions are as accurate as possible thanks to the work of the following contributors:

Barbara Richey

Ben Carter

Billy Fields

Christine Sheeran

Cindy Dickerson

Elton Clark

Franz Gimmler

Frederick Schaedtler

Gene Olig

Graham Stroh

Heather Deutsch

Jennifer Kaleba

Jessica Leas

Jessica Tump

Kelly Cornell

Lorili Toth

Marianne Fowler

Meghan Taylor

Ryan Phillips

Sarah Shipley

Rails-to-Trails Conservancy would like to give special thanks to the Tawani Foundation and American Express Company for their generous support that helped make this guidebook possible.

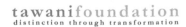

INDEX

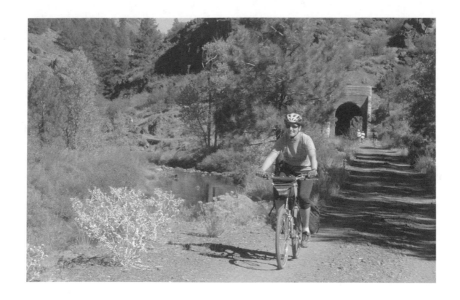

Become a member
of Rails-to-Trails Conservancy

As the nation's leader in helping communities transform unused railroad corridor into multi-use trails, Rails-to-Trails Conservancy (RTC) depends on the support of its members and donors to create access to healthy outdoor experiences.

You can help secure the future of rail-trails and enhance America's communities and countryside by becoming a member of Rails-to-Trails Conservancy today. Your donations will help support programs, projects and services that have helped put more than 13,000 rail-trail miles on the ground.

Every day, RTC provides vital technical assistance to communities throughout the country, advocates for trail-friendly policies at the local, state and national level, promotes the benefits of rail-trails and defends rail-trail laws in the courts.

Join RTC in *"inspiring movement"* and receive the following benefits:

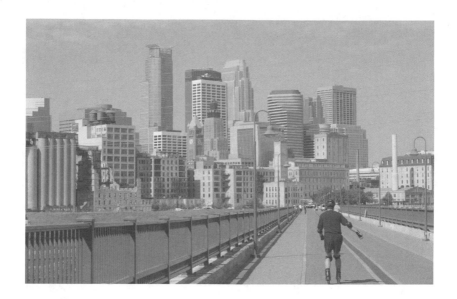

❶ New member welcome materials including *Destination Rail-Trails*, a sampler of some of the nation's finest trails

❷ A **subscription** to RTC's quarterly magazine, *Rails to Trails*.

❸ **Discounts** on publications, apparel and other merchandise including RTC's popular rail-trail guidebooks.

❹ The **satisfaction** of knowing that your dollars are helping to create a nationwide network of trails.

Membership benefits start at just $18, but additional contributions are gladly accepted.

Join online at **www.railstotrails.org**

Join by mail by sending your contribution to Rails-to-Trails Conservancy, Attention: Membership, 1100 17th St. NW, 10th Floor, Washington, DC 20036.

Join by phone by calling 1-866-202-9788.

Contributions to Rails-to-Trails Conservancy are tax deductible to the full extent of the law.

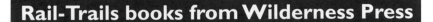